Childhood Depression

The *Journal of Children in Contemporary Society* series:

Childhood Depression

Theodore A. Petti, MD
Editor

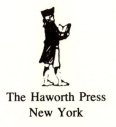

The Haworth Press
New York

Childhood Depression has also been published as *Journal of Children in Contemporary Society,* Volume 15, Number 2, Winter 1982.

The Haworth Press, Inc., 28 East 22 Street, New York, NY 10010

Library of Congress Cataloging in Publication Data
Main entry under title:

Childhood depression.

    "Childhood depression has also been published as Journal of children in contemporary society, volume 15, number 2, winter 1982"—Verso t.p.
    Includes bibliographies.
    1. Depression in children. I. Petti, Theodore A.
RJ506.D4C47 1983   618.92'8527   83-58
ISBN 0-917724-95-X

Childhood Depression

Journal of Children in Contemporary Society
Volume 15, Number 2

CONTENTS

TREATMENT

EPIDEMIOLOGY

ADVANCED RESEARCH

WILLIAM ISLER, *Advisor, Early Childhood Education, Bureau of Curriculum Services, Department of Education, Harrisburg*

MARSHA POSTER ROSENBLUM, *Director, Carnegie-Mellon University Child Care Center, Pittsburgh*

JUDITH RUBIN, *Art Therapist, Pittsburgh Child Guidance Center, Pittsburgh*

ETHEL M. TITTNICH, *Adjunct Assistant Professor, Program of Child Development and Child Care, School of Health Related Professions, University of Pittsburgh*

Introduction

Problems are often dramatized in the literature long before they are recognized as contemporary social issues. Around 1887, Thomas Hardy was concerned about depressed children. In his novel, *Jude The Obscure,* one such character was a little boy nicknamed Little Father Time, "because I looked so aged, they say." After Little Time lived the early part of his childhood with his maternal grandparents in Australia, he was returned to England to live with his father, Jude, and his father's mistress, Sue. Both of them had a genuine compassion and concern for Little Father Time.

Adverse social, economic, and health circumstances forced them to relocate several times. When Jude was quite ill and living by himself, Sue, Little Time, and their two children were evicted from their little room. The landlord wouldn't have children kicking the walls in the halls. Late on a rainy night, Sue and Little Time wandered into the streets to locate a new lodging, but after every householder looked askance at both of them, the little boy had misgivings about being born and said, "I ought not to be born, ought I?" And in his continued reflective mood added, "I think that whenever children be born that are not wanted they should be killed directly, before their souls come to 'em, and not allowed to grow big and walk about." Sue then felt it was time to confide in him that there would soon be another baby in the family. Little Time's reaction was one of sorrow and he replied while weeping and sobbing, "How ever could you, mother, be so wicked and cruel as this when you needn't have done it till we was better off, and Father well . . . "

The following morning, while Jude was visiting Sue, he heard Sue shriek from the closet where the children slept. To his horror, he saw his two children hanging from garment hooks by a piece of box-cord and Little Time hanging on a nail in a similar fashion. On the floor, a note was found which was written by the boy with a lead pencil he carried: "*Done because we are too menny.*"

In this classic story, Little Father Time is a symbol of all children who have suffered many losses and grieve their existences.

After years of debate, and almost 100 years after Hardy wrote about Little Father Time, a growing number of specialists in the medical profession are concluding that children can suffer from depression. Prior to this time, many clinicians felt children could not suffer depression because they had not yet matured to a neurological developmental level where they could be depressed or it was not recognized as it manifested itself differently from that as observed in adults. Now, it is estimated that in this country, there may be over 40,000 children who are suffering varying degrees of depression.

For the past decade, there has been a growing body of literature that establishes the existence of childhood depression, there are newly designed instruments for its identification and measurement, and there are newly developed therapeutic modalities used for treatment. The collection of articles within this issue focus on the current status of childhood depression as it relates to the still existing conflicts and controversies over diagnosis, depression and dysphoria in the preschool child, the assessment of childhood depressions, areas of stress causing depression, intervention and prevention strategies, and in conclusion, future trends in the study and treatment of childhood depression.

We are honored and privileged to have this comprehensive collection of articles written by those who are nationally recognized as having made significant contributions to children with disturbing behaviors. We acknowledge their efforts with deep gratitude.

MIF

OVERVIEW

Controversy and Conflicts in Childhood Depression

Elva Orlow Poznanski, MD

ABSTRACT. Childhood depression has had in the past, and still has many controversies, the first being whether it existed at all. Even now, child psychiatrists feel uncomfortable with the concept of depression in childhood and with this, the implication of misdiagnosis. Pediatricians who have always used a medical model of illness have less difficulty with the existence of depression in children. Pediatricians in the recent past faced a similar predicament with the acknowledgment of the existence of child abuse. This diagnosis, like childhood depression, was missed for decades.

Parents, much more than doctors, often have trouble handling the thought that their child may be depressed, let alone suicidal. But then, parents have always had difficulty accepting any serious illness with their offspring, especially psychiatric illness. Clinically, the group who are the most honest, and most accurate in recognizing depressive behavior in themselves and others have been children. Children, rather than their parents give the best description of their feelings, especially in the affective disorders.

The Denial of the Existence of Childhood Depression

Depression in children was not recognized for decades, as children were, for the most part, regarded as incapable of experiencing depression. The myth of childhood being a happy carefree state

Elva Orlow Poznanski is Professor of Psychiatry at the University of Illinois and Director of the Youth Affective Disorders Clinic, 912 South Wood Street, Box 6998, Chicago, Illinois 60680.

(despite literary giants who described it differently) apparently pre-judiced the observations of the public and psychiatry. Rie (1966) states that "the familiar manifestations of adult, nonpsychotic depression are virtually nonexistent in childhood" (pp. 653-685). Adults may have experienced a twinge of jealousy that children could escape the responsibilities of adulthood, i.e., children did not have reasons to be depressed. Since depression could not occur in children, reasons had to be found to explain this phenomenon. The rationales for this viewpoint were multiple: that children lacked an adequate superego development (Rochlin, 1965); that they lacked experience with separations until the end of adolescence (Wolfen-stein, 1966).

The Concept of "Masked Depression" or "Depressive Equivalents"

In the 1960s, the concept of masked depressions (Glaser, 1967; Lesse, 1974) or depressive equivalents (Toolan, 1962) was put forth. This concept held that the depressive affect was not directly expressed except for possibly short periods of time and that a variety of behavioral problems were alternate ways of expressing depres-sion in childhood and adolescence.

The concept of masked depression in children evolved from the bereavement literature, which likely had the same biases in their observations of bereaved children as those who observed childhood depression. The normal reactions of children to bereavement are still less known than those of adults. Children have been described as expressing less affective grief than adults. Wolfenstein (1966) speaks of the "short sadness span" of children, referring to her perception that children cannot tolerate prolonged states of sadness and anger. Furthermore, Wolfenstein theorized that in bereavement in children, the depressive affect is isolated from thoughts of death.

At any rate, children in response to the death of a parent or sib-ling, do demonstrate periods of sadness though they are thought to be of shorter duration than is characteristic of the adult. What has been recognized, is the children who have suffered a significant loss, can have disturbed behavior for long periods of time. Because the affective component was not comprehended but a wide variety of behavioral disturbances appeared such as temper tantrums, disobedience, truancy, running away from home, and accident pro-neness, the idea that children show "depressive equivalents" rather than demonstrating open depressive affect was the first concep-tualization of depression in children (Toolan, 1962).

In the 1960s the concept of masked depressions was used as the mode of expression of depression in children. Glaser (1967) wrote on "masked depression in children and adolescents." He felt masked depression could be the underlying cause of many behaviors including delinquency, school phobias, and learning difficulties. In 1967, a special edition of the *Journal of the American Psychiatric Association* dealt with depression. The single article on depression in children described it only in terms of "masked depression" (Glaser, 1967).

Toolan (1962) used the term "depressive equivalents" and felt a wide variety of symptomatology could act as depressive equivalents such as psychosomatic symptoms, eating and sleeping disturbances, boredom, restlessness, etc. Since depressive equivalents were not directly tied to an affective state almost all of childhood psychopathology could be viewed as "depressive equivalents." Retrospectively, however, many of the case histories of children thought to have depressive equivalents gave, in fact, good descriptions of a depressed child. The difficulty appears to have been in recognizing the affective state.

There were at least three difficulties with accepting depressive equivalents as a predominant view of depression in childhood: (a) it assumed that depressive affect is only rarely observable in children, (b) the behaviors cited as expressing "equivalents" to depression were so diverse as to encompass most of the nonpsychotic psychopathologies in children and adolescents, and (c) the linkage of such conditions to depressive affect was frequently tenuous or nonexistent. Clearly from clinical and research experience the concept of depressive equivalents as the mode of expressing depression in childhood is unacceptable.

The Recognition of Depressive Affect in Children

An exception to the general trend in the 1960s was the work of Sandler and Jaffe (1965) from the Hampstead Clinic who examined the psychoanalytic records of 100 children and set forth 9 features which they felt were commonly associated with depressive affect. Their paper was concerned, primarily, with theoretical formulations. However, it constituted an important step forward because the authors were very clear in stating that depressive affect *is* seen in children.

The early 1970s produced a dramatic shift in the thinking about childhood depression in this country and in Europe. In 1970 Poznanski and Zrull (1970) published a clinical study of 14 children who showed recognizably overt depression. Malmquist (1971) wrote an extensive review of the literature of childhood depression that was well integrated with his own theoretical concepts. There was the implicit and at times, uncomfortable inference that children can become depressed. Also in 1971, the Fourth Congress of the Union of European Pedopsychiatrists convened in Sweden and took as its theme, "Depressive States in Childhood and Adolescence." Cytryn and McKnew (1972, 1974) published two articles on childhood depression; one on classification and a second on possible biochemical correlates. Again in 1972, the GAP Committee on Child Psychiatry published a report and included for the first time, a category of childhood depression under psychoneurotic disorders in a proposal for a diagnostic nomenclature suitable for children and adolescents. At last childhood depression was admitted to exist and it was possible to find it listed in at least one system of diagnostic nomenclature for children.

Depressive Affect versus Depressive Syndrome in Children

There is now fairly widespread acceptance of the existence of depressive affect in children. Two papers, Carlson and Cantwell (1980) in "Unmasking Masked Depression in Children and Adolescents" and Cytryn, McKnew and Bunney (1980) acknowledge that overt depression is seen in children and that the mask had been on the observers rather than on the children.

A current controversy centers around the issue of whether a primary depressive syndrome occurs in children that is analogous to a Major Depressive Disorder in Adults. Somehow, even the possibility of endogenous depression in children causes disbelief in some professionals. Actually, many times the issue is not depression in children but whether one group of children should be treated under "the medical model." Some professionals feel threatened by the word depression as they feel it implies treatment by M.D. as opposed to Ph.D. or M.S.W. However, this paper is not intended as a format for that conflict.

When depressive affect was first recognized, the behaviors felt to coexist with depression varied widely with different authors. Each researcher in the early and mid 1970s in childhood depression, including the author of this paper used idiosyncratic groups of symptoms in describing childhood depression. Kovacs and Beck (1977) reviewed nine authors' sets of symptomatology in which the number of symptoms listed varied from five to seventeen. Since 1975, most clinical researchers have moved to tighten their diagnostic criteria. There is now greater unanimity in the diagnostic criteria used in clinical research as compared with the status five years ago.

The majority of professionals engaged in clinical work do not use diagnostic criteria in the assessment of children who may be depressed. This is unfortunate because any of the currently used diagnostic criteria is better than no diagnostic criteria. There is a widespread tendency to go from completely ignoring depression in children to suddenly labeling all dysphoric affect in children as representing a depressive syndrome.

Weinberg (1973) was the first researcher to specify diagnostic criteria prior to diagnosing a group of children as depressed or nondepressed. He also treated these children with tricylitic medication. When this paper was published, the editors felt compelled to preface it with a note that the editors didn't necessarily agree with Weinberg's article. One assumes that such disagreements between editors and authors are common and that the need to print a statement of this nature underscores the emotions and conflict that article engendered.

Weinberg's criteria have been used in both modified and unmodified form. While his criteria were specifically designed for children, the original model came from Feighner's Criteria (1972). Some researchers have used the two sets of adult criteria, i.e., Research Diagnostic Criteria (RDC) (1972) and the Diagnostic and Statistical Manual of Mental Disorders (DSM III) (1980), in the unmodified form for their research in childhood depression. Poznanski (1979) uses her own criteria derived from the data analyses of moderately and severely depressed children. Actually all four sets of criteria are amazingly close and the two sets of criteria specific for children, i.e., Weinberg's and Poznanski's, are similar to those of DSM III and RDC.

The major objection for the use of DSM III criteria or RDC criteria is that they have been used unmodified from adults in the diagnosis of children. The controversy centers on diagnostic criteria with the argument frequently expressed that children should not be treated as little adults. The problem which is more central to the diagnosis of depression in children is not diagnostic criteria but rather the difficulty of recognizing the form of the cardinal depressive behaviors in children. The developmental stage of the child determines the coloration of the content. For example, a depressed child may go to school complaining, doesn't do much schoolwork in the classroom, may daydream, looking out the window and/or fight with classmates. An adult may drag himself/herself to work, do a sloppy job at work and behave in an aloof and irritable manner with the other employees. Both may be showing a depressed mood and have difficulty concentrating, but the clinical pictures are so vastly different that the similarities can become obscured. Behavior needs to be observed by unbiased eyes. These are difficult prerequisites and account for many of the conflicts and controversies in all areas of psychiatry.

The classification of depression in adult psychiatry has sparked considerable controversy. The split into bipolar versus unipolar illness has appeared to be the most solid division for adult affective disorders but this is of little help in child psychiatry where manic-depression illness is rare. The possible existence of mania in children is controversial. Many psychiatrists report that manic-depressive illness appears with puberty and that the only rare exception is a late latency aged child. Others contend that the prejudice against labeling a child's affect as depressed has shifted and now includes a reluctance to label other affective states in children, i.e., euphoria. Other classifications of the vast array of depressions in adults has been problematic, with some arguing in favor of splits such as primary-secondary, reaction-nonreaction, etc. While others feel depression is unidimensional and any divisions are, therefore, arbitrary. Since the classification of depression in adults except for the bipolar-unipolar distinction is an issue which has not yet been resolved, it would appear premature to impose the arguments pro and con for depression in children.

Several classification systems, specifically for children, have been proposed. None have gained universal acceptance. Malmquist (1971) was one of the first, his is primarily theoretical and while it provided a well organized model, it bore little relation to clinical realities. Others, like Cytryn and McKnew (1972), have devised a classification system derived from a clinical base, but the classification does not indicate either treatment strategies or possible prognosis.

Theories about etiology directly influence treatment approaches regardless of the lack of any information about either etiology or treatment. Thus psychoanalytically inclined therapists recommend outpatient psychotherapy exclusively for children with genetically transmitted mood disorders, such as bipolar illness, while biologically inclined therapists are inclined to think solely in terms of the use of medication. Some therapists feel drug therapy in children for any purpose is practically tantamount to child abuse while others want to use the latest drug treatment in any refractory problem with a child. The arguments pro and con for drug therapy with children with affective disorders are almost totally irrational. They are based on political ideology acquired prior to recognizing depression in children. Tricylitics medication in children, in doses comparable to that used in adults for depression, i.e., more than the prescribed dose in enuresis, have not been sufficiently tested in children to know if they work and if they are safe. One cannot assume that antidepressant medication will have the same effect in depressed children as in depressed adults. The antipsychotic group of drugs should have taught us that lesson. Any special modifications of psychotherapy including cognitive approaches have yet to be described for depressed children. Thus treatment in depressed children has barely started to be explored.

The denial of affect has had a long and venerable history in psychiatry. Although one of the major tasks of psychotherapy is to link feelings with events, the study of affect as such, has largely been avoided. Freud's theory of development centers around psychosexual maturation while Piaget focuses almost exclusively on cognition. A general theory which includes the development of affect has yet to be put forth. Meanwhile increased knowledge about pathological mood states in children will enhance our knowledge about childhood depression and pave the way for study of normal affect in children. Increased knowledge usually reduces conflict and controversies.

REFERENCES

Carlson, G., & Cantwell, D. Unmasking masked depression in children and adolescents. *American Journal of Psychiatry*, 1980, *137*, 445-449.

Cytryn, L., & McKnew, D. H. *American Journal of Psychiatry*, 1972, *129*, 149.

Cytryn, L., & McKnew, D. H. *Archives of General Psychiatry*, 1974.

Cytryn, L., McKnew, D., & Bunney, W. Diagnosis of depression in children: A reassessment. *American Journal of Psychiatry*, 1980, *137*, 22-25.

Diagnostic and Statistical Manual of Mental Disorders. erd ed. Washington, D.C., American Psychiatric Association, 1980.

Feighner, J. P., Robins, E., Guz, S. B., Woodruff, R. A., Winokur, G., & Munoz, R. Diagnostic criteria for use in psychiatric research. *Archives of General Psychiatry*, 1972, *26*, 57-63.

Glaser, K. *American Journal of Psychotherapy*, 1967, *21*, 565-574.

Group for the Advancement of Child Psychiatry. *Psychopathological disorder in childhood*, Report #62, New York, 1972.

Kovacs, M., & Beck, A. T. An empirical approach towards a definition in childhood depression. In J. G. Schueterbrandt & A. Raskin (Eds.), *Depression in children: Diagnosis, treatment and conceptual models.* New York: Raven Press, 1977.

Lesse, S. Depression masked by acting-out behavior patterns. *American Journal of Psychotherapy,* 1974, *28,* 352-361.

Malmquist, C. *New England Journal of Medicine,* 1971, *284,* 887-893.

Poznanski, E., & Zrull, J. *Archives of General Psychiatry,* 1970, *23,* 8-15.

Poznanski, E., Eook, S. C., & Carroll, B. J. A depression rating scale for children. *Pediatrics,* 1979, *64,* 442-450.

Rie, H. *Journal of American Academy of Child Psychiatry,* 1966, *5,* 653-685.

Rochlin, G. *Griefs and Discontents.* Boston: Little, Brown & Co., 1965.

Sandler, J., & Jaffe, W. G. *International Journal of Psychoanalysis,* 1965, *46,* 88-96.

Toolan, J. M. *American Journal of Orthopsychiatry,* 1962, *32,* 404-414.

Weinberg, W., Rutman, J., & Sullivan, L. Depression in children referred to an educational diagnostic center. *Journal of Pediatrics,* 1973, *83,* 1064-1072.

Wolfenstein, M. *Psychoanalytic Study of the Child,* 1966, *21,* 93-123.

Depression in the Preschool Child

Javad H. Kashani, MD, FRCP(C)

ABSTRACT. There are no systematic studies which deal primarily with the investigation of depression among preschool age children. At the present time, there is controversy about the existence of depression as a clinical entity in this age group. DSM III uses diagnostic criteria for depression in preschool children which are modified from the criteria used in prepubertal, adolescents and adults. This paper discusses contributory factors, symptomatology, epidemiology, assessment and intervention in preschool children with depression and concludes with a description of the unique feature of depression in this age as contrasted with other age groups.

The term depression may denote a symptom (i.e., feeling sad, unhappy, blue, or down, in short—dysphoria). In this article, however, the term depression refers to a clinical syndrome which, in addition to dysphoric mood, also entails other symptoms, i.e., disturbances of appetite and weight, insomnia and changes in activity level, which remain over a period of weeks rather than a very short period of time. Although a temporary episode of dysphoric mood due to environmental factors is frequent in the preschool child, this is entirely distinct from depression as a diagnostic entity.

Depression as a clinical syndrome has not yet been systemically investigated in preschool children. In infants, however, Spitz (1946) has described "anaclitic depression." He found that children separated from a maternal figure after the age of six months demonstrated not only persistent crying and an apathetic attitude with immobile facies, but also a poor appetite and sleep disturbances, with slowed reactions to physical stimuli. These symptoms parallel closely those of depression in adulthood. Gaensbauer (1980) reported anaclitic depression in a three and one-half month old in-

---

Dr. Kashani is Associate Professor of Child Psychiatry, University of Missouri–Columbia. Reprint requests should be directed to the author at 3 Hospital Drive, Columbia, Missouri 65201.

fant who showed sad facies, apathy, withdrawal, psychomotor retardation and loss of pleasure.

Controversy surrounds the question of the existence of depression in the preschool child. Some investigators feel that depression in children under 5-6 years of age either doesn't exist or is extremely difficult to diagnose (Kovacs and Beck, 1977). These authors cite the work of Piaget and his co-workers as support for their position since facility of language communicative skills doesn't develop until around the age of 7 years. Other studies support the existence of depression in the preschool child both theoretically (Weiner, 1975) and clinically (Poznanski and Zrull, 1970; and Paulson et al., 1980). Weiner believes that since attachment to important adult figures begins at 6-8 months of age and that disturbed behavior results from loss of contact with that figure, it is theoretically possible that depression exists at virtually any stage in the developmental sequence. Clinical investigations of Poznanski and Zrull also support the existence of depression in preschool-aged children. They have described children as young as three years in whom disturbances of appetite, failure to gain weight, lack of affection for any persons, and withdrawal were prominent. In Frommer's study (1972) of depressed preschool children reduction of appetite, abdominal pain and sleep disturbances with accompanying anxiety were typical symptoms. Katz (1979) described the depressed preschool child to have an overall mood of sadness, unhappiness, or irritability. The children in the study appeared withdrawn, bored, discontented, not easily satisfied, and with little capacity for enjoyment. In addition to sleep and appetite disturbances, rocking and other repetitive activities with bursts of overactivity also were characteristic of these children.

Contributory Factors

Loss is the most consistently reported feature of depression. This, of course, encompasses an extremely broad category. It may include an obvious physical loss in the child (e.g., loss of a limb, Kashani et al., 1981), or a loss referable to the child's environment. A loss of physical health or physical deformity (e.g., major burn) could contribute to depression by depriving the child of playmates, rejection by peers and/or parents, with the subsequent loss of self-esteem. The loss as well may be environmental, such as separation from parents (or parental surrogates) to whom the child has developed a dependent attachment. Whether due to death, chronic illness, separation or divorce within the family, its impact may be similar. The loss may include not only parents, but also for example, an involved grandmother or babysitter. Albeit, less dramatic than physical loss, a parent's sudden loss of involvement with the child, whether a result of parental illness or the birth of a new sibling, could also severely impact the child. Another issue related to loss involves the issue of parental deprecation and rejection. Many depressed children have felt rejected by their parents or caretakers, either overtly (constant fault-finding, or neglect) or more subtly, lack of interest in the child's activities. Explanations for this rejection may lay with the parent's own type and degree of psychopathology, especially depression. In fact, the existence of parental depression is the most consistent finding in depressed children. As a result of this depression, the parent may become withdrawn, neglectful, and even abusive. However, it is not yet clearly understood how depression in the parents affects the child; the child may, for instance, identify with the depressed parent, or adopt parental coping mechanisms into his/her own personality. Another unanswered issue involves the role of genetic predisposition in the child and his parents. To date, it remains unclear if any or a combination of these factors may be of etiologic significance in the development of depression in these youngsters.

The preschool child, due to his total dependence on a caretaker, is particularly more vulnerable to the loss of a parental figure than his prepubertal or adolescent counterpart. Parental views and opinions of him will have a tremendous impact on the formation of his self-concept. The adolescent and prepubertal child, on the other hand, have peers as another resource for gratification and perhaps even dependence, but for the preschool child, parents and parental surrogates are the most important (and often the only) source of gratification.

Symptomatology

Although several recent articles have described depression in prepubescent children, adolescents and adults according to basically similar criteria (Puig-Antich et al., 1979; Cantwell and Carlson, 1979; Carlson and Cantwell, 1980; Kashani et al., 1981), these guidelines cannot be generalized to preschool children. Accordingly, even the American Psychiatric Association's latest edition (1980) of diagnostic and statistical Manual of Mental Disorders for children under six years of age, listed below, are different from that of other age groups.

a. Dysphoric mood that may have to be inferred from persistently sad facial expressions,
b. In addition to the above, at least three of the four following:
   1. Poor appetite or failure to gain expected weight;
   2. Disturbances of sleep (insomnia or hypersomnia);
   3. Hypoactivity (rather than hyperactivity);
   4. Loss of interest and seeming indifference to immediate surroundings (apathy).

Epidemiology

No single study to date has studied depression among preschool children utilizing a relatively well-accepted set of criteria such as DSM III. Some of the studies have suffered either from a lack of well-defined and widely accepted diagnostic criteria (Frommer, 1972), or poor stratification according to age groups (Pearce, 1978). As a result, at the present time, the exact frequency of depression among preschool children is not accurately known. Poznanski and Zrull (1970) reported that of 1788 children seen in the outpatient department at University of Michigan, 14 children under 12 years of age were found to be overtly depressed; and that three of these children were under six years of age. Paulson et al., (1978) from a sample of 662 children aged 4-12 years seen at UCLA, identified 34 severely depressed children, of whom five were under six years of age.

Assessment

Parents and relatives may provide complementary diagnostic data for the diagnosis of depression in adolescents; however, the patient remains the primary source of information. In the prepubertal child, the main source of information is still the patient, and the contribution of parents, teachers, and others assumes greater significance if complete evaluation and a firm diagnosis is to be obtained and the importance of multiple source of information has been stressed (Kashani et al., 1981). The assessment of preschool children, however, differs from that of all other age groups. For instance,

DSM III requires a sad facial expression rather than verbal expressions of sadness as a diagnostic criterion. Disturbances of appetite and sleep are also based on observation of the child in different times and settings. Hypoactivity is also observed, rather than related by the patient. Finally, apathy and indifference (to toys, candies, etc.) are also best evaluated by observation. Two main differences then segregate depression in the preschool child from that in prepubertal children, adolescents and adults: (1) diagnosis is based on observation rather than verbalization; and (2) symptoms are most frequently reported by adults, e.g., parents, relatives and nursery personnel. In considering the latter, some difficulties might expect to be encountered. For example, it may be difficult for some parents (or other caretakers) to judge or interpret accurately the child's facial expressions; accordingly, inaccurate observations are expected occasionally. Along these lines, it would seem prudent to observe, if possible, the interaction between the child and his caretaker(s). Although the observation of parent-child interaction is extremely helpful at any age, during the preschool period, a careful assessment of this dyad relationship becomes perhaps even more critical due to the child's limited communicative skills. Therefore, a conjoint interview (observing the child and parent together) during which this interaction can be assessed, may serve to support or refute parental reports. Furthermore, this may also uncover either overt or covert rejection, neglect, and/or lack of interest in the child. In summary, the process of assessment in the preschool child is indeed unique and different than in all other age groups.

Intervention

A thorough assessment and evaluation of the depressed preschool child may provide us with some insight toward possible contributory factors. Once identified, intervention may be directed toward removal of these factors. For instance, in a child with depression whose mother is also severely depressed, parental treatment may have an indirect therapeutic benefit on the child as the mother may become more capable of meeting the child's needs. Or again, given a loss for which there is a potential substitute, providing that substitute may effectively relieve some of the depressive symptoms.

Generally, the younger the child, the more responsive he is to environmental changes; therefore, parental counseling becomes the treatment of choice (Cytryn and McKnew, 1980). Just as, then, the diagnostic criteria of depression in preschool children are specialized, so also treatment of the very young child via manipulation of the environment is unique to this age group. The importance of improving the child's self-concept through providing success even in minor events should be stressed to the parents; similarly, accentuating the child's assets and positive aspects, rather than finding fault, should become a matter of routine. In essence, therapy comprises the removal of known causative factors, most of which usually stem from environmental causes.

Conclusion

There is controversy concerning the existence of depression in preschool children. At the same time, a systematic investigation of depression among preschool children is lacking, due at least in part to a lack of consensus on acceptable criteria. This article describes some of the unique features of depression among preschool children in contrast to prepubertal children, adolescents and adults. Salient points concerning depression in this age group include:

1. Diagnostic criteria characteristic of this age group should be utilized;
2. Observation as a method of assessment assumes much more importance than verbalization in this age group;
3. Treatment includes both members of the dyad (child and parent); in the very young child and the treatment of choice comprises parental counseling.

Based on the above, the preschool depressed child should not be grouped together with depressed prepubertal children and adolescents. Furthermore, an immediate research need entails investigation of the frequency of depression among preschool children both within the general population, as well as within selected clinic samples.

REFERENCES

Cantwell, D. P., & Carlson, G. A. Problems and prospects in the study of childhood depression. *Journal of Nervous and Mental Disorders,* 1979, 522-529.

Carlson, G. A., & Cantwell, D. P. Unmasking masked depression in children and adolescents. *American Journal of Psychiatry,* 1980, *137,* 445-499.

Cytryn, L., & McKnew, D. H. Affective disorders. In H. I. Kaplan et al. (Eds.), *Comprehensive Textbook of Psychiatry III.* Baltimore: Williams and Wilkins, 1980, 2798-2809.

Diagnostic and Statistical Manual of Mental Disorders of American Psychiatric Association (DSM III), Third Edition, 1980, 213-214.

Frommer, E. A., Mendelson, W. B., & Reid, M. A. Differential diagnosis of psychiatric disturbance in preschool children. *British Journal of Psychiatry*, 1972, *121*, 71-74.

Gaensbauer, T. J. Anaclitic depression in a three-and-one-half-month-old child. *American Journal of Psychiatry*, 1980, *137*, 841-842.

Kashani, J., Barbero, G. J., & Bolander, F. Depression in hospitalized pediatric patients. *Journal of American Academy of Child Psychiatry*, 1981, *20*, 123-134.

Kashani, J., Husain, A., Shekim W. O., Hodges, K. K., Cytryn, L., & McKnew, D. H. Current perspectives on childhood depression: An overview. *American Journal of Psychiatry*, 1981, *138*, 143-153.

Kashani, J., Venzki, R., & Millar, E. A. Depression in children admitted to hospital for orthopedic procedures. *British Journal of Psychiatry*, 1981, *138*, 21-25.

Katz, J. Depression in the young child. In J. Nowells (Ed.), *Modern Perspectives in the Psychiatry of Infancy*. New York: Brunner, Mazel, 1979, 435-449.

Kovacs, M., & Beck, A. T. An empirical-clinical approach toward a definition of childhood depression. In J. G. Schulterbrandt & A. Raskin (Eds.), *Depression in Childhood: Diagnosis, Treatment and Conceptual Models*. New York: Raven Press, 1977.

Paulson, M. J., Stone, D., & Sposto, R. Suicide potential and behavior in children age 4 to 12. *Suicide Life Threat Behavior*, 1978, *8*, 225-242.

Pearce, J. B. The recognition of depressive disorder in children. *Journal of the Royal Society of Medicine*, 1978, *71*, 494-500.

Petti, T. A. Depression in hospitalized child psychiatry patients. *Journal of American Academy of Child Psychiatry*, 1978, *17*, 49-58.

Poznanski, E., & Zrull, J. P. Childhood depression: Clinical characteristics of overtly depressed children. *Archives of General Psychiatry*, 1970, *23*, 8-15.

Puig-Antich, J., Perel, H., Lupatkin, W., Chambers, W. J., Shea, C., Tabrizi, M. A., & Stiller, R. L. Plasma levels of Imipramine (IMI) and Desmethylimipramine (DMI) and clinical response in prepubertal major depressive disorder: A preliminary report. *Journal of American Academy of Child Psychiatry*, 1979, *18*, 616-627.

Spitz, R. Anaclitic depression. *Psychoanalitic Study of the Child*, 1946, *2*, 113-117.

Weiner, I. B. Depression in Adolescence. In F. F. Flach & S. C. Draghi (Eds,), *The Nature and Treatment of Depression*. New York: John Wiley and Sons, 1975.

ASSESSMENT

The Assessment of Depression in Young Children

Theodore A. Petti, MD

ABSTRACT. The assessment of depression in the infant, pre-school and early school age child is described. A variety of scales and interviews which are of potential use to the caretakers of young children are reviewed. The role of evaluation in caring for children with depression is stressed: beginning with awareness of the disorder; of methods to assess and monitor the depression; and of the need to understand the total picture of the child who is suffering from the depression.

INTRODUCTION

As we become more aware of depression and its effect on children, the assessment of this disorder becomes increasingly important. Assessment of the depressed child is a multifaceted task. It requires the following: an awareness of depression as a significant disorder; knowledge of how depression manifests itself through the developmental sequence from infancy to adolescence; familiarity with scales and rating instruments which provide a depression or related factor; and an orientation toward detailing the contributions from home, neighborhood and school which culminate in the depres-

Dr. Theodore A. Petti is Assistant Professor of Child Psychiatry, University of Pittsburgh School of Medicine and Director, Section on Children and Youth, Office of Education and Regional Programming, Western Psychiatric Institute and Clinic, University of Pittsburgh, 3811 O'Hara Street, Pittsburgh, Pennsylvania 15261.

sion. A thorough assessment is an essential prerequisite for the clinician/caretaker to have as a basis for developing sufficient insight into the depressive phenomenon and for then intervening in a meaningful and constructive manner.

This paper will describe the assessment of young children particularly those age 8 and under. The varied clinical aspects of depression in children are richly depicted elsewhere in this journal issue and will be supplemented to help clarify the assessment issues.

Assessment of Depression in Infants

Cases describing infants suffering from anaclitic depression have been reported from ancient times (Langdell, 1973). Early descriptions were predominantly anecdotal and descriptive. Actual rating scales to assess depression in infants are not available. However, the diagnosis can be made by determining the presence or absence of the classic symptoms of anaclitic depression as elaborated by Spitz (1946). The following behaviors generally occur during or after ages 6 to 8 months and following 4 to 6 weeks of separation or lack or nurturance from the mother:

— Apprehension and sadness, to weepingness
— Decreased contact with caretakers and rejection of the environment to withdrawal
— Retardation of development, and dejection, to stupor
— Loss of appetite and refusal to eat, to loss of weight
— Sleeplessness and insomnia

Bowlby (1961) has placed these and other observations into a fairly standard sequence of occurrence for children between 6 months and 6 years of age: Protest, Despair and Detachment. In the Protest phase, the young child responds to loss or separation by anger and tears with behaviors indicating a demand and hope for mother's return. This phase alternates with the Despair phase which follows and consists of a quieting in behavior and a presumed yearning for the absent mother. The Detachment phase then follows in which the child seems to forget about the mother and even at her return, the child seems neither to be interested nor to recognize her. Tantrums and episodes of destructive or violent behavior occur through all three phases.

In assessment it is important to recognize the phase in the Protest-

Despair-Detachment continuum to which the depressed infant has progressed. Phillips (1979) poignantly and succinctly describes a 9-month-old infant who had entered into the Detachment phase: unresponsive, difficult to arouse, withdrawn and undernourished. He also highlights the importance of assessing the "Caretaker Problems and Life Events" which are particularly critical for the young child or infant: parental depression (usually the mother) which leads to rejection, abuse/neglect (physical and/or psychological), and incapacity/inability to provide parenting (mothering), separation from the parenting figure, and chronic illness. O'Brien elaborates more fully on this issue.

Diagnosing depression in infants and assessing the extent of the process and contributing factors are crucial for reversing the process and minimizing the long-term damage. The importance of recognizing depression in infants, understanding the dynamics of the situation and then developing appropriate interventions has been classically described by Bakwin (1942). Infants and children in the pediatric service of Bellevue Hospital were noted to develop a disproportionate amount of infections, failure to thrive and unexpectedly poor response to treatment. Bakwin observed that they looked like depressed, little old men. The intervention of having them held more regularly during the day appreciably reversed the problematic behaviors.

Assessment of Depression in the Preschool Child

The presentation of depression in the preschool child has been comprehensively described by Kashani in this issue; he notes that no well accepted criteria have been employed in studying these children and that their assessment is unique compared to older children or adolescents. Like the infant, the 2 to 6 year old has difficulty verbalizing depressive affect and cognitions. Observation of the toddler and preschooler is very important in assessment. Some scales which screen for maladaptive or psychopathologic behavior in children do have subscales or factors which relate to depression.

For example, the Behavioral Screening Questionnaire of Richman and Graham (1971) is a 60-item interview schedule for use in learning about the development, health and behavior of 3-year-olds. Some of the 12 scales of behavior include eating, sleeping, mood, and relationship to siblings or peers. Information is gathered by means of an interview with the parent. In contrast the Children's

Behavior Checklist (Arnold and Smeltzer, 1974) can be filled out by parents or parent surrogate. For children in the 2 to 12 year age range, factors such as withdrawal/depression, somatic complaints and inattentive unproductiveness have been found. However, this instrument may not be helpful in actually identifying depressed children (Petti, 1978).

A scale of potential usefulness in hospital, nursery and day care settings is the Children's Behavior Inventory (CBI) of Burdock and Hardesty described elsewhere (Petti, 1978). Subscales of lethargy/dejection and self-depreciation are weighed toward depression. The items are divided into age groups of 1 to 3 years, 3 to 5 years, 5 to 7 years up to 13 to 15 years. The CBI discriminates well between normal and emotionally disturbed children and staff of Headstart, Day Care, nursery schools or related agencies can be trained in its use. The symptom checklist (Kahn and Rosman, 1973) can also be completed by teachers or other caretakers. It is a 58-item list of behaviors which have two major dimensions or factors (Interest-Participation vs. Apathy-Withdrawal and Cooperation-Compliance vs. Anger-Defiance) for children ages 3 to 6 years.

Another instrument that might be helpful and has been used in a number of settings is the Child Behavior Checklist (Achenbach, 1979). This is a 130-item scale which is completed by the parent(s) or primary caretaker and details most of the symptoms and strengths found in children. This scale is particularly helpful in detailing social competence by requesting information regarding quality and degree of activity in social activities, interpersonal behavior with peers, sibs and parents, and academic performance. The 113 behavior items are rated for the past year as very true, somewhat true or not true. The beauty of this approach is that a profile can be determined through scoring either by hand or computer. This provides an overview of the child's behavior, clusters strengths and problems and compares the results to those of children of the same sex and age group. These normative values have been completed for ages 4 to 5, 6 to 11, and 12 to 16 years. Some of the profiles or clusters include depression, somatic complaints and social withdrawal. A diagnosis of depression cannot be made using this instrument but a great deal of information regarding strengths and weaknesses can be obtained for use in planning interventions and possibly in assessing, over time, how successful the interventions may have been.

The Quincy Behavior Checklist (QBC) is a scale which offers

promise in assessing relevant behaviors of depressed preschool children; but it is in the process of still being developed (Orvaschel et al., 1980). The QBC is a 38-item scale which can be filled out by parents or school personnel for 4 to 5 year olds. Included in the 11 areas of social/emotional dysfunction which QBC taps are Depression, Social Withdrawal, Apathy/Lack of Initiative, and somatic complaints.

These instruments have been presented in order to provide the reader with exposure to published scales of potential use to the person in the "front line" working with young children. Further descriptions and comments on most of these scales are provided elsewhere (Orvaschel et al., 1979). As we enter an era where everything we do will potentially require review, having access to standardized scales may prove extremely useful in meeting such a mandate.

We will now sidestep briefly from the quantitative approach to look at observational and descriptive assessments of preschool children experiencing the separation and divorce of their parents. Wallerstein and Kelly (1975) provide us a good example of this approach. They have studied the responses of children from 2-½ years to teenagers to events which are prototypical of the loss type events generally associated with the development of depression.

The response of nine very young preschoolers (ages 2-½ to 3-¾ years) were followed for one year after an initial evaluation. Three of these children were found to exhibit an actual worsening of their clinical condition on the follow up visit. Wallerstein and Kelly describe in detail how one of these children, a 3-year-old boy at the time his parents went through the turmoil of separation and divorce, had developed a "consolidated childhood depression" by the time of reevaluation. They attribute the worsening of clinical condition in the three young preschoolers to the breakdown in functioning of the caretakers and the severe impairment of their capacity to parent.

Using the effects of parental divorce as a natural and expected stimulus for childhood depression, the efforts of these careful investigators provide us means to assess the depression and its roots in the middle (3-¾–4-¾ years) and older (5-6 years) preschoolers. Wallerstein and Kelly report that more than half of the middle preschool group had worsened in clinical condition at the one year follow-up evaluation. Movement toward greater inhibition and constriction in their fantasy, play and behavior was noted along with decreased self-esteem and increased sadness, neediness, and anxiety.

These changes were believed related to prior psychiatric difficulties reported for most of the fathers. These men had also been involved in unrealistic demands and harsh punishment; many improved after the divorce, while the mothers became more distant. Thus these children were faced with complicated and changing relationships with their parents, which made the integration of what had happened in their lives very difficult. The importance of the father in the assessment process, even if not in the home, should be underscored.

The description of these children and those who fared better provides a model for how one might go about assessing and following the course of children experiencing a significant loss and/or disruption in their lives—from parent report, interview with the child, play and language, and school report.

Similarly, in the oldest preschool group, more than a third were worse on follow-up: "the behaviors and preoccupations of these vulnerable children were consolidating into childhood depression of varying intensities and pervasiveness." The youngsters at the initial assessment were noted to demonstrate acute unhappiness, anxiety, denial, and inability to think about the divorce, various symptoms and depressive feelings. The greatest impact on these children over time was seen in school performance and social functioning. School reports documented high restlessness, excessive daydreaming, fears of failure, and distractibility. Their increase in aggressive behavior was paralleled in their fantasy themes of burning and exploding houses and undoing the father's departure. Thus it is clear that depression or depressive symptomatology of varying degrees is present in these preschool children and that both quantitative and qualitative approaches to their assessment can be instituted.

Assessment of Depression in the Young School Age Child

The psychiatric literature is more detailed regarding the approaches to assessing depression in the young school age child. McConville for example does a beautiful job of describing the affective type of depression in the 6 to 8 year old and has developed a scale to screen for or measure it. The scale (McConville et al., 1973) is based on a 15-item questionnaire which relies heavily on the verbal productions of children in a residential setting. Its focus on the developing child and high interrater reliability are genuine assets. It may not be useful in evaluating or measuring changes in children seen on an outpatient basis or in acute care facilities. Petti (1978) has described a number of approaches to diagnosing and measuring depression in school age children and presents a critical review of the literature related to the use of specific criteria or scales.

The Children's Affect Rating Scale (Cytryn and McKnew, 1979) also provides the observer with an assessment instrument operating within the conceptual framework of development. It attempts to quantify fantasy productions, behavior and verbalizations for children 6 to 12 years of age.

The diagnostic criteria for assessing depression in adults have been reproduced in a structured interview which has been useful for research work. Puig-Antich and Associates (1978) have modified this scale for use with children, ages 6 to 17 years. Both the child and parents are interviewed by trained personnel and diagnoses ranging from Major Depression, Separation Anxiety, Conduct Disorder and Schizophrenia may be derived. This scale might prove difficult to use in a clinic or school setting, but should prove of great utility where precise research is being conducted.

The Bellevue Index of Depression (Petti, 1978) is another useful interview schedule for children. It is a modification of a scale by Weinberg and Associates (1973) which has been employed in assessing children with academic and school related behavior problems. This is a semi-structured interview. The child and parents are interviewed separately regarding 10 major areas, including: Dysphoria, Self-Deprecatory Ideation, Agitation/Hostility, Sleeping and Eating Problems; Socialization; Energy and Interests, and School Attitudes and Behavior. Employing this scale, which correlates highly with clinicians impression of moderate to severe depression, allows both the child and the parent to respond to non-threatening questions regarding suicidal ideation and behavior, depression and related behaviors. The parents can be given a paper-pencil form to complete rather than an interview. The format for interviewing 6 to 12 year old children has suggested questions to be used to elicit the data for each item. This scale has been particularly useful to this author in assessing the depth of depression and in following the course of children seen on an outpatient or partial hospital program basis. The original Weinberg scale is less specific, but has been reported as useful in selecting children who are likely to respond to antidepressant medication treatment.

As with the preschooler, it is important to know how the school age child is responding to his/her environment at home and at school, to learn about the fantasy life of the child and about the home conditions. School is an important variable for such children, and an understanding of potential learning or social problems in that setting are crucial. Since depression, dysphoria or extreme sadness can occur as a response to a variety of situations and happenings, it is important to assess the degree of dysphoria and its contribution to any other problems. Moreover, many early school age children have attentional difficulties and/or over activity and these difficulties must be evaluated regarding their role in the depressive picture.

The differential must be made between a child with an attentional problem with resultant depression versus a child responding to a depression by becoming hyperactive and inattentive. Phillips (1979) notes that for 6 to 8 year olds, depressive symptoms include school refusal, aggression, learning problems, hyperactivity and a variety of affective symptoms. A good history and observation of the child can assist in determining whether the depression is primary or secondary. Rating scales described above may be of some assistance in this task. Examples addressing these issues and demonstrating how the assessment process and treatment planning can be integrated for young children have been presented elsewhere (Petti, 1981,1982). Physiologic indices for diagnosing depression in children will be discussed later in this journal.

Summary

The basic approach to assessing the child who is experiencing significant depression consists of:

1. Being aware of the disorder
2. Using assessment instruments and strategies that are geared to the age of the child, the type of children you work with and the needs that you have for planning intervention strategies, and
3. Understanding the whole child and his/her dynamics
   a. the internal psychic organization of the child, including fantasy and preoccupations/worries
   b. the cognitive strengths and weaknesses which can be used to understand and/or correct problem areas for the child
   c. the level of academic functioning as it relates to (b)
   d. the social skills and adaptive behaviors used or available to the child or which may be needed by the child to function

e. the family and social environments which have contributed to the depression and/or which can be used for treating the depression

f. the internal physiology of the child—including chronic or acute disease and possible physiologic changes accompanying the depression.

The treatment of depressed children is made easier once an understanding of the above factors has been gained through the assessment process.

REFERENCES

Achenbach, T. M. The Child Behavior Profile: An empirically based system for assessing children's behavior problems and competencies. *International Journal of Mental Health,* 1979, *7,* 24-42.

Arnold, L. E., & Smeltzer, D. J. Behavior checklist factor analysis for children and adolescents. *Archives of General Psychiatry,* 1974, *30,* 799-804.

Bakwin, M. Loneliness in infants. *American Journal of Diseases of Children,* 1942, *63,* 30-40.

Bowlby, J. Childhood mourning and its implications for psychiatry. *American Journal of Psychiatry,* 1961, *18,* 481-498.

Cytryn, L., & McKnew, D. H., Jr. Affective Disorders. In J. D. Noshiptz (Ed.), *Disturbances in Development of the Basic Handbook of Child Psychiatry.* New York: Basic Books, Inc., 1979.

Kohn, M., & Rosman, B. A two factor model for emotional disturbance in the young child: Validity and screening efficacy. *Journal of Child Psychology and Psychiatry,* 1973, *14,* 31-56.

Langdell, J. Depressive reactions of childhood and adolescents. In S. A. Szurek & I. M. Berlin (Eds.), *Clinical Studies in Childhood Psychoses.* New York: Brunner Mazel, 1973.

McConville, B. J., Boag, L., & Purohit, A. P. Three types of childhood depression. *Canadian Psychiatric Association Journal,* 1973, *18,* 133-137.

Orvaschel, H., Sholomskas, D., & Weissman, M. M. The assessment of psychopathology and behavioral problems in children: A review of scales suitable for epidemiologic and clinical research. (1967-1978). NIMH Series AN No.1, DHHS Publication No. (ADM) 80-1037, Washington, D.C., 1980.

Petti, T. A. Depression in hospitalized child psychiatry patients: Approaches to measuring depression. *Journal of the American Academy of Child Psychiatry,* 1978, *17,* 49-59.

Petti, T. A. Active treatment of childhood depression. In J. F. Clarkin & H. I. Glazer (Eds.), *Depression: Behavioral and Directive Intervention Strategies.* New York: Garland Press, 1981.

Petti, T. A. Depression and withdrawal in children. In T.H. Ollendick & M. Hersen (Eds.), *Handbook of Child Psychopathology.* New York: Plenum Publishing Corp., 1982. 1982.

Phillips, I. Childhood depression: Interpersonal interactions and depressive phenomenon. *American Journal of Psychiatry,* 1979, *136,* 511-515.

Puig-Antich, J., Blau, S., Marx, N., Greenhill, L., & Chambers, W. Prepubertal major depressive disorder: A pilot study. *Journal of the American Academy of Child Psychiatry,* 1978, *17,* 695-707.

Richman, M. & Graham, P. A behavioral screening questionnaire for use with three-year-old children. Preliminary findings. *Journal of Child Psychology and Psychiatry,* 1971, *12,* 5-33

Spitz, R., & Wolf, K. M. Anaclitic depression: An inquiry into the genesis of psychiatric conditions in early childhood. *Psychoanalytic Study of the Child,* 1946, *2,* 313-342.

Wallerstein, J. S., & Kelly, J. B. The effects of parental divorce: Experiences of the preschool child. *Journal of the American Academy of Child Psychiatry,* 1975, *4,* 600-616.

Weinberg, W. A., Rutman, J., Sullivan, L., Penick, E. C., & Dietz, S. G. Depression in children referred to an educational diagnostic center: Diagnosis and treatment. *Pediatrics,* 1973, *83,* 1065-1072.

Depressive Themes
in Children's Fantasies

Elaine S. Portner, PhD

ABSTRACT. Puppet stories were elicited spontaneously from 65 school children between the ages of eight and nine in a recent study designed to collect normative data. Findings provided an opportunity to study more closely a subgroup within the population: those children who deviated significantly from the norm, most notably in their preoccupation with misfortune. This paper will discuss (1) techniques of child assessment through play, (2) research efforts, (3) findings of the normative study, and (4) depressive themes among the clinically suspect subgroup.

Educators and clinicians alike have sought ways to identify what is normative among the behavior and expression of children. Educationally, such knowledge enables school planning to relate effectively to normal development. For clinicians, expectations form a basis for studying deviations from the norm. Achievement scores and IQ tests provide standardized measurements of learning and academic potential. Other methods are used to assess the child's emotional world. Behavior checklists, parent, teacher, and self-reports contribute to a complete diagnostic picture. However, a most articulate expression of children occurs through their symbolic play.

Definitions of play vary among theorists and therapists. Regardless of the orientation there seems to be general acknowledgement of play as a unique expression of the individual. The growth of the field of play therapy has promoted respect for play as the work of childhood and as the child's natural mode of communication. As early as the 1930s, Murray (1936) posited that "the investigation of fantasy should be included in every examination of personality that

Elaine S. Portner is Assistant Professor of Psychiatry at the University of Pittsburgh School of Medicine, and Family Therapy Coordinator of the Adolescent/Young Adult Module at Western Psychiatric Institute and Clinic. Reported findings are part of research conducted for her doctoral dissertation, *A Normative Study of the Spontaneous Puppet Stories of Eight Year Old Children,* University of Pittsburgh, 1981.

29

aims to be thorough" (p. 115). Ekstein (1966) stated that whatever the patient produces, acts out, plays out, or talks out is, in effect, a communication of the unconscious conflict. By the time children are three or four, they should be able to project themselves in fantasy expression (R. Gould, 1972); by the time they reach latency, the capacity to engage in dramatic play ought to be well established (Sarnoff, 1976).

TECHNIQUES OF ASSESSMENT THROUGH PLAY

Techniques have been developed specifically to elicit play or fantasy material from adults and children in a diagnostic testing situation. These procedures incorporate the use of projection in which people react to stimuli by endowing responses with their own idiosyncrasies (Frank, 1948). The spontaneity inherent in a play technique circumvents resistance by enabling people to present symbolic material of often unspeakable concerns.

The Rorschach was the first major clinical and research instrument and spearheaded the projective techniques movement (Beck, 1937). Many have reported the use of a patient's drawings in therapy (Appel, 1931; Machover, 1949; Naumberg, 1947). Because children's stories are believed to be akin to dreams and free associations in the adult, they often accompany the diagnostic and therapeutic repertoire (Ames, 1966; Freud, 1928; Klein, 1932; Levy, 1939). Approaches vary in the manner of eliciting stories, including picture cards (Bellak, 1949), fables (Despert, 1946), and mutual storytelling (Gardner, 1969).

The use of puppets in clinical work with children has been described by many (Bender & Woltmann, 1936; Hawkey, 1951; Howells & Townsend, 1973; Irwin & Shapiro, 1975). Puppet play "makes possible the interchange of reality and fantasy worlds by using 'make believe' characters" (Woltmann, 1964, p. 324). The appeal of puppets encourages engagement with the task, while the choices made among characters and themes provide valuable information for both clinical and research purposes.

RESEARCH EFFORTS

Previous investigations of expressive play and fantasy have recognized the richness of the information available. But research studies often have suffered from a variety of limitations. A major difficulty has been the size and selective nature of most samples studied. In general, samples have been too small and have not been sufficiently representative with regard to important background characteristics. Nor have data analyses adequately measured the comparative impact of such variables.

Recently, research was conducted to overcome these limitations by collecting normative data from 65 latency age children of diverse backgrounds (Portner, 1981). The specific aim was to ascertain the typical form and content of the spontaneous puppet stories of eight year old children, and to understand the differences in form and content as they relate to several potentially important background variables: sex, race, socioeconomic status, school achievement, self-concept, and history of family disruption.

The procedure replicated part of the dramatic play interview in a study of traumatized children (Elmer, 1977), in which examiners encouraged children to select puppets and create a spontaneous drama, using a technique developed by Irwin and Shapiro (1975). A closer look at the spontaneous puppet stories of the children in the Elmer (1977) study revealed a preponderance of themes of misfortune (Irwin, Portner, Elmer, & Petti, 1981). However, those children, both traumatized and matched controls, were found to be notably impaired and maladjusted in several measures, results thought to be consequences of their low socioeconomic status. The normative study (Portner, 1981) was conducted to provide a baseline by which to assess children of this age in general and to contribute to the understanding of the earlier findings.

NORMATIVE FINDINGS
AMONG EIGHT-YEAR-OLD CHILDREN

Spontaneous puppet stories were elicited from 65 eight-year-old school children (29 boys and 36 girls), 72% white, distributed across all social classes. Stories were audiotaped, transcribed, and rated, using criteria reflective of the author's psychodynamic orientation.

Overall findings indicated that most children at age eight readily create a story, incorporating four puppet characters and addressing three to four themes. Children were usually able to conceptualize a moral for their story, congruent with its meaning. In general, sex differences had significantly more impact on outcomes than other background characteristics.

Girls tended to produce stories with positive affective tone and prosocial themes of nurturance and sociability. Boys created stories that were generally negative in affective tone, while telling stories with primarily aggressive themes. Contrasted with boys, girls tended to demonstrate more maturity, affectively and cognitively, as evidenced in greater empathy and problem-solving skills. Two sample stories from the normative study (Portner, 1981) are representative of the findings.

Story Sample 1: The Smart Monkey

Jack told a story that is characteristic of those typically told by boys. It is primarily an unelaborated narrative report of action, rather than an interactional dialogue. Reasonably coherent, it contains a clever, if magical, solution to a difficult problem, in which the underdog wins.

> One day the monkey was in his tree until the tree started to shake. There was a wolf after a rabbit. The rabbit was running very fast. The wolf stared at the monkey. The monkey started to run, but the wolf soon got to him. The monkey was still running when the, when the wolf grabbed the tail.
>
> He said, "I surrender, I surrender. Eat me if you please."
>
> So the monkey climbed a tree like he had some . . . like you got an axe, chopped the tree down on the wolf, and the wolf never ate a rabbit or monkey again.

He named the story "The Smart Monkey" and identified the monkey as his favorite "for being so smart to knock down the tree." The following congruent moral was offered by Jack: "Never go near a smart wolf—or a wild dog!"

Sample Story 2: The Maid that Never Wanted to Do Anything

Although Jack's story was sparse, other stories from both sexes contained dialogue, rather than simple narrative, and were more elaborate in content. Judy's story is such an example.

> One day the king came in and sat in his crown and he said, and the girl was out playing and his little princess was out playing

on the lawn and she fell and her arm got hurt and the king ran out and then he, and he called the nurse.

The nurse came out and said: What happened?

King: She was out playing and she fell.

Nurse: Oh, let me see her arm. It looks like it's broken to me.

King: Oh, okay. What will we have to do?

Nurse: Well, could you call the royal servant?

King: Servant! Servant!

Servant: Yes.

King: Could you go to, um, the town and get some bandages?

Servant: Yes I will.

And he rode off on his horse.

Then the maid that never wanted to do anything ran and she said: You know what? I have to do Everything in this castle. I have to make the food, wash the dishes, dust, and do everyting else. And I think it's no fair that I have to do all the work.

King: Well, you just go do a couple more things and I'll see if I can get somebody.

Maid: Okay.

And then the servant came back and said: Here are your bandages.

King: Okay, I'm going to go in and get the nurse.

The nurse came in and said: Thank you. I will take this.

And she took them over and she wrapped the princess' arm up with the bandages. She went over to the king and said: I fixed her arm.

And the king came out and said: Oh, thank you very much. For that you can come and have tea with me today.

Judy's drama demonstrates nurturing, protection, and empathy, complete with romance and a happy ending, all of which are typical of girls' stories according to the normative findings. Fantasy royal family characters are included in Judy's story which addresses everyday grievances of overwork and injury, while incorporating humor. Her favorite character was an entertaining and complaining maid. The moral of her story, "Help each other," is indicative of problem-solving qualities which she demonstrated.

DEPRESSIVE THEMES AMONG A CLINICALLY
SUSPECT SUBGROUP

Among the 65 children of the normative study, there is a subgroup of children, boys and girls, whose story characteristics are conspicuously different from the normative findings. Contrasted with the reported expectations of children's fantasy presentations of this age, those children who deviated from the norm seen clinically suspect. This group includes children who, unlike the norm, identify with the role of the victim and are preoccupied with themes of misfortune. Perseveration of story themes and rigidity of roles are prevalent among this group. Characteristics of their fantasies suggest emotional disturbance, reminiscent of the findings of traumatized children and controls studied earlier (Elmer, 1977; Irwin et al., 1981). The subgroup of the present population which defies the normative categories represented 14% of the subjects, a frequency consistent with the reported incidence of clinical maladjustment among children in the general population (M. S. Gould, Wunsch-Hitzig, & Dohrenwend, 1980).

The clinical expression of the depressive process in children can be manifested in many ways. Cytryn and McKnew (1974) considered three factors: fantasy manifestation of depression, verbal expression of depression, and mood and behavior. Of these, they found fantasy manifestation of depression to occur in nearly all diagnosed depressed children. Using a variety of projective tests, they noted the following themes: mistreatment, thwarting, blame or criticism, loss and abandonment, personal injury, death and suicide. They found that children were less apt to talk directly about their depression, and that their observable mood and behavior were even less reliable diagnostically. Both hyperactivity and aggressiveness were reported to be among the mood and behavior manifestations which masked depression. On the other hand, the fantasies of the children provided most significant diagnostic data.

Paradoxically, very depressed children may have a difficult time fantasizing. Petti (1978) noted that despite the seemingly universal occurrence of depressive themes in the stories of depressed children, "the fact that fantasy material cannot be elicited from a child may be a prime indicator of the depth of the depression the child is experiencing" (Petti, 1978, p. 52). He cautioned that scales and other methods of assessment should correlate with a clinician's judgement concerning the presence or absence of depression in order to make a valid diagnosis.

Social class may confound a diagnosis of depression, particularly in assessments which require a verbalization. The Hope Scale (Gottschalk, 1974), for example, requires that an individual speak spontaneously about an interesting or dramatic life experience. Studies have demonstrated that low SES children have limited verbal skills (Miller & Gerard, 1979) and diminished capacity to use fantasy to express aggression (Eichler, 1972) compared to middle or upper class children. Since a significant proportion of diagnosed depressed children are culturally and socioeconomically underprivileged (Petti, 1978), it remains a challenge to differentiate whether sparse verbalization from a child is a reflection of social class or indicative of depression.

The 65 children of the normative study readily participated in the request to produce a story, regardless of social class. The puppets were sufficiently appealing and the procedure adequately supportive to enable even the most constricted or limited among the group to produce a fantasy. Following are two sample stories of children whose fantasies aroused suspicion of maladjustment because of recurrent or exclusive depressive themes of misfortune.

Story Sample 3: Mister Rogers

Tony produced a story that was incoherent and chaotic, requiring continuous attempts by the examiner to clarify the confusion.

> Okay. This wolf be out in the forest. The boy, he be walking. Then wolf come down and he says "RRRRRRR." He might have bite, he might have bite him in the leg. Then they kill him. Might bite him in the neck. And then he strangle him. He strangle him. And then he take him, he take him. Maybe he could take him and give him some, give some to his other family . . .

> (The wolf takes the boy to feed him to his wolf family)

> Yeah. He's the mother. He going to get him. Take this to him. He takes it here with him. He says, "See our dog be taking stuff" Then they put him down. They put him down and they

eat him. Eat him all up. Then all the wolf dies and he, he gets all sick. He gets and this big one gets sick. And then so he dies, too. That's the end.

Tony, when asked to explain the death of the wolves, reported that they died because they ate the boy's brain. He named the boy "King Friday" and called the story "Mister Rogers," which refers to the most nonthreatening and reassuring of children's television programs, serving as a defense mechanism for Tony to deny the frightening content he has produced. The story reflects a perseveration of mutilation, destruction, and death.

Story Sample 4: The Lost Children

Tammy created a story, mostly narrative, in which vulnerability and a confusing sense of unpredictable danger were pervasive.

Two little boys and girls took the dog for a walk. Okay. And so this man, somebody came and messed with them. So they hurried to get their dog and scared him away. So when they got home, they told their mother and father.

So they said, "Your son and your daughter was picking on my children".

And so, and so they all of them went to the movie. The father was in a car. He went to warm up the car. So the mother, she cooked dinner. And then, when they eat they went out to the movie. They were full and then they ate some more. And then they were hugging and they was looking at the movie. And then the girl and boy was still talking about that. Then the dog, the dog came to stay home. It was hungry and it was, and somebody broke into their window and opened it so the dog was chasing after them. They had a gun and they killed the dog. And then when the mother and the father and the two little girls and boys . . . came back, they went in the house and then they went to sleep.

And then the murderer came again and tried to take the little boy and the little girl. So the little boy and the little girl was frightened and then in the morning they didn't see their dog, so they was crying. They, and then them two was out back playing, playing hopscotch, no they was playing ring-around-the-rosey. And they kissed each other cause they thought the dog wasn't dead. And then when they found out they started crying. They tried to find him. They tried to find their dog. And they got kidnapped, they got kidnapped.

Tammy ended the story abruptly. She named it "The Lost Children," preferring to be the mother rather than the children because "the mother can beat the kids." She offered two morals to the story: "Not to run away" and "keep your windows locked." Life's rewards (food, movies) and hardships (death, robbery, kidnapping) all seem to occur unexpectedly, in a world in which children and dogs are not safe.

SUMMARY

Children of the clinically suspect subgroup, like Tony and Tammy, offer stories in which danger befalls the helpless, with no apparent rescue in sight. The preponderance of themes of misfortune and victimization mark the children as distinctively depressive in their fantasies. Likewise, the population of the Elmer (1977) study, notably impaired and maladjusted, was preoccupied with fantasy themes of injury and loss, ideas most associated with feelings of being a victim.

Interestingly, normative findings from the present study (Portner, 1981) reflect an absence of victims as preferred identifications by boys or girls, who also commonly tend to avoid themes of misfortune. These findings corroborate studies reported by Maccoby and Jacklin (1974) who observed that boys and girls, through most of the school years, do not see themselves as victims.

The results of the work described in the present article confirm (1) the effectiveness of the puppet interview to generate fantasy data from children regardless of background, (2) the reliability of the procedure to obtain normative data, and (3) the subsequent capacity to identify depressive components in the presentation of children.

REFERENCES

Ames, L. B. Children's stories. *Genetic Psychological Monograph*, 1966, *73*, 337-396.

Appel, K. E. Drawings by children as aids to personality studies. *American Journal of Orthopsychiatry*, 1931, *1*, 129-144.

Beck, S. J. Introduction to the Rorschach method: A manual of personality study. *American Orthopsychiatric Association Monograph*, 1937.

Bellack, L. *The TAT and CAT in clinical use*. New York: Grune & Stratton, 1954.

Cytryn, K., & McKnew, D. H. Factors influencing the changing clinical expression of the depressive process in children. *American Journal of Orthopsychiatry*, 1974, *131*, 879-881.

Despert, J. L. Psychosomatic study of fifty stuttering children. *American Journal of Orthopsychiatry*, 1946, *16*, 100-113.

Eichler, J. M. *A developmental study of action, fantasy and language aggression in latency aged boys*. Doctoral dissertation, Boston University, 1972.

Ekstein, R. *Children of time and space, of action and impulse*. New York: Appleton-Century-Crofts, 1966.

Elmer, E. *Fragile families, troubled children: The aftermath of infant trauma*, Pittsburgh: University of Pittsburgh Press, 1977.

Frank, L. K. *Projective methods*. Springfield, Illinois: Charles C. Thomas, 1948.

Freud, A. *Introduction to the techniques of child analysis*. New York: Nervous and Mental Disease Publishing Co., 1928.

Gardner, R. A. Mutual storytelling as a technique in child psychotherapy and psychoanalysis. *Science and Psychoanalysis*, 1969, *14*, 123-136.

Gottschalk, L. A. A hope scale applicable to verbal samples. *Archives of General Psychiatry*, 1974, *30*(6), 779-785.

Gould, M. S., Wunsch-Hitzig, R., & Dohrenwend, B. P. Formulation of hypotheses about the prevalence, treatment, and prognostic significance of psychiatric disorders in children in the United States. In B. P. Dohrenwend, B. S. Dohrenwend, M. S. Gould, B. Link, R. Neugebauer, & R. Wunsch-Hitzig (Eds.), *Mental illness in the United States*, New York: Praeger Publishers, 1980.

Gould, R. *Child studies through fantasy*. New York: Quadrangle Books, 1972.

Hawkey, L. The use of puppets in child psychotherapy. *British Journal of Medical Psychology*, 1951, *24*, 206-214.

Howells, J. G., & Townsend, D. Puppetry as a medium for play diagnosis. *Child Psychiatry Quarterly*, 1973, *6*, 9-14.

Irwin, E., Portner, E., Elmer, E., & Petti, T. *Joyless children: The effects of abuse over time*. Paper presented at the International Congress of the American Society of Psychopathology of Expression, Boston, April, 1981.

Irwin, E. C., & Shapiro, M. I. Puppetry as a diagnostic and therapeutic technique. In I. Jakab (Ed.), *Psychiatry and Art* (Vol 4.). Basel, Switzerland: S. Karger, 1975.

Klein, M. *The psychoanalysis of children*. London: Hogarth Press, 1932.

Levy, D. Release therapy. *American Journal of Orthopsychiatry*, 1939, *9*, 713-736.

Maccoby, E. E., & Jacklin, C. N. *The psychology of sex differences*. Stanford, California: Stanford University Press, 1974.

Machover, K. *Personality projection in the drawing of the human figure*. Springfield, Illinois: Charles C. Thomas, Inc., 1949.

Miller, B. C., & Gerard, D. Family influences on the development of creativity in children: an integrative review. *The Family Coordinator*, 1979, *28*, 295-312.

Murray, H. A. Techniques for a systematic investigation of fantasy. *Journal of Psychology*, 1936, *3*, 115-143.

Naumberg, M. Studies of the 'free' art expression of behavior problem children and adolescents as a means of diagnosis and therapy. *Nervous & Mental Disorders Monograph*, New York: Coolidge Foundation, 1947.

Petti, T. A. Depression in hospitalized child psychiatry patients: approaches to measuring depression. *Journal of the American Academy of Child Psychiatry*, 1978, *17*, 49-59.

Portner, E. S. *A normative study of the spontaneous puppet stories of eight year old children*. Unpublished doctoral dissertation, University of Pittsburgh, 1981.

Sarnoff, C. *Latency*. New York: Jason Aronson, Inc., 1976.

Woltmann, A. G. The use of puppets in understanding children. *Mental Hygiene*, 1940, *24*, 445-458.

Woltmann, A. G. Psychological rationale of puppetry. In M. R. Haworth (Ed.), *Child psychotherapy.* New York: Basic Books, Inc., 1964.

CHILDREN UNDER STRESS

Dysphoria in Children with Severe Burns

Frederick J. Stoddard, MD
Karen G. O'Connell, MEd

ABSTRACT. This is a descriptive article, defining dysphoria in the burned child, and focusing on the specific stressors which relate to its development in severely burned children. Attention is given to the following factors: physiological pain and its management, separation and hospitalization, and losses incurred. The three stages of burn care are briefly described. Case material is presented to illustrate the management of dysphoria at each of these stages. The importance of an interdisciplinary team approach is emphasized. The probability for successful adjustment of the severely burned child is discussed. Implications for further research are presented.

The purpose of this paper is to provide descriptive, clinical information based on our experiences with young burned children. It is not intended to be a research paper. Indeed, having reviewed three data bases, ERIC, *Psychological Abstracts,* and *Index Medicus,* in search of material on this topic, we found nothing. To the best of our knowledge this is the first article specifically dealing with dysphoria in young burned children. Three illustrative cases are presented.

Frederick J. Stoddard is Director of Psychiatry, Shriners Burns Institute, Boston, and Clinical Associate in Psychiatry, Massachusetts General Hospital. Karen G. O'Connell is a doctoral student in Counseling Psychology and Special Education Administration, Boston College. Reprint requests should be directed to: Dr. Stoddard, Shriners Burns Institute, 51 Blosson Street, Boston, Massachusetts 02114.

SCOPE OF THIS PROBLEM

Ten thousand children in this country are severely burned every year. Seventy percent of this group is under five years of age. Burns are the third leading cause of accidental death during childhood (Herrin & Crawford, 1972). In the United States where many of the homes are wooden structures, the percentage of burn injuries sustained in house fires is very high. Among young children there are two types of common burns. Scald burns often occur when toddlers, curious about the environment and wishing to explore, pull cups of hot coffee off tables or grab pot handles protruding from the stove. The result is a burn involving multiple areas of the body. Electrical burns are also frequent. They occur when youngsters crawling around on the floor chew on electric cords. In 1980 the Boston Unit of the Shriners Burns Institute admitted 86 acute patients. Of this number 60 were eight years or under. These statistics represent a typical year.

The Shriners Burns Institute in Boston is a thirty-bed, teaching hospital serving both acutely burned children and those returning for reconstructive procedures. The part-time mental health staff is composed of a psychiatrist and a psychologist, each of whom conducts weekly groups for the patients; two social workers, who see families regularly; and trainees in the above mentioned disciplines. An after-care nurse has also joined the staff.

Overview

Psychological reactions to severe burn trauma cover a wide variety of affects. Concomitants of a serious burn may include: tremendous pain, loss of limbs, loss or permanent impairment of one or more bodily functions, severe scarring and disfigurement, and loss of loved ones. When we speak of dysphoria as it relates to the burned child, we mean a mood state manifesting itself in eating or sleep disturbances, especially nightmares, sad facial expression, psychomotor retardation, withdrawal, excessive tearfulness, and a lack of appropriate reactivity to pain. This dysphoria may constitute both an adaptive response to overwhelming trauma and a developmental interference. While a burned child often experiences anxiety states, bouts of anger, and aggression, we do not include them in our discussion of dysphoria per se, even though they are sometimes related.

The dysphoria we see in the vast majority of burned children relates to a variety of transient stressors. According to D.S.M. III (American Psychiatric Association, 1980), these children are diagnosed as having post-traumatic stress disorders, as the stressor, the burn trauma "evokes significant symptoms of distress" and "is generally outside the range of usual human experience." Many burned children also experience brief organic affective syndromes, mainly deliria. At present we do not have data on the specific frequencies.

A few children suffer from primary affective disorders, and manifest chronic signs of depression. As yet we have not needed anti-depressants in the treatment of children under age eight. We find this group to have many risk factors predisposing them to a depressive episode. They are: genetic factors, particularly depression in and/or loss of a parent; a history of previous losses; a disorganized family situation prior to the burn injury; and a family unable to adapt to the sequelae of the burn trauma. Given a stable adaptive family structure and a child who has experienced few pre-burn psychological difficulties, the likelihood of dysphoric mood to persist appears minimal.

The specific stressors which relate to the development of dysphoria in severely burned children are:

1. *Physiological.* Organic affective syndromes such as deliria, autistic withdrawal and hallucinoses, may be provoked by neurotoxicity secondary to smoke inhalation, metabolic changes, medications and their interactions (e.g., opiates, chloropromazine, and haloperidol), sepsis, cardiorespiratory distress, or post-operative syndromes. Sensory deprivation and/or overstimulation of the child in intensive care is another common cause. Little has been written about these syndromes in children (Antoon et al., 1972, Murray, 1978).
2. *Pain.* The burned child must cope with two types of pain. Physical pain from the injury and from treatment, especially dressing changes, and emotional pain caused by bodily disfigurement, fear of death, etc. (Stoddard, 1981).
3. *Separation and hospitalization.* The severely burned child is always hospitalized, often placed in a BCNU (bacteria controlled nursing unit) where he/she is isolated from parents and subjected to strange procedures, frightening machines and people in masks and gloves (Bransetter, 1969).

4. *Loss.* The burned child often loses several of the following: control of bodily functions, limbs, parents, siblings, pets, or personal possessions and previous body image (Stoddard, 1980).

Children and families are seen for crises intervention work upon acute admission and around amputations, death, etc. Most of the clinical work done directly with patients on an individual basis is short-term ego supportive therapy aimed at supporting adaptive defenses and lessening the interference caused by maladaptive ones.

In developing children, the management of dysphoria must take into account the child's cognitive level, primary modes of communication, and predominant affects. For example, an acutely burned infant, refusing food, and suffering from insomnia will not benefit from careful explanation of what is going to be done during his/her dressing change, but will respond positively to being touched or held by mother or a consistent caretaker.

A major portion of our time is spent providing support and consultations to staff, many of whom must inflict pain on patients via dressing changes and physical therapy, and many of whom work intensely with the critically ill child hovering between life and death. Providing an opportunity for staff to express their feelings about their work and providing support and concrete suggestions is a necessary part of life on a burn unit (Bernstein, 1976).

STAGES OF BURN CARE AND ASSOCIATED DYSPHORIC SYMPTOMS: CASE ILLUSTRATIONS

For the purpose of organization we will divide the psychological care of the burned child into three phases. The first phase is the acute, lasting from several days to several weeks. During this period the crucial issue is life or death. The child is often isolated in a BCNU, suffers great pain, and is connected to some form of life support system. The primary dysphoric symptoms seen during this stage are eating and sleep disturbances, lack of reactivity to pain, psychomotor disturbance, and a turning away from caretakers.

The following is an example of an acutely burned child manifesting signs of dysphoria.

Case I: Acute Phase

Kevin is a 14-month-old boy who sustained second and third degree burns to 30% of his total body surface area. The burns were located on his face, hands, chest and legs. These burns were incurred as the result of a housefire. His four-year-old sister was also hospitalized with less serious burns. The origin of this fire is unclear. No adult was present in the home at the time.

Kevin was placed in a BCNU upon admission, and we observed acute psychomotor symptoms of dysphoria not previously present, i.e., extreme restlessness, constantly kicking his legs, relaxation of muscles around the mouth resulting in frequent drooling and eyes "rolling back" in his head; attentional disturbances, i.e., withdrawal from mother and staff and constant focusing upon his left hand; eating disturbances i.e., refusal to eat; lack of reactivity to any pain; and periods of inconsolable, fretful crying not related to any pain-inducing procedure. Neurological examination failed to reveal a specific cause of the disturbance but physiological factors were likely contributors.

After a short period of time Kevin began to take some nourishment, more from his mother than from staff. His psychomotor disturbances improved. He became calmer and stopped drooling and rolling his eyes. A transitional object (a stuffed animal from home) had been placed in his unit as well as a mobile. Gradually he began to focus on them instead of his hand. Kevin's lack of reactivity to pain, sorrowful crying and refusal to utter any of the simple words he had learned continued.

As his medical condition improved, Kevin was able to come out of the BCNU onto the open ward. At this juncture rapid improvement could be seen. Kevin was now held and rocked a great deal by his mother and several of the nurses who consistently participated in his care. As a result he began to make more speech-like sounds and would say "hi," "no," and "mama."

Kevin's case is a good example of how dysphoric symptoms associated with acute burn trauma disappear in a young child who heals quickly.

The second or intermediate phase of burn care lasts from the end of the acute phase until discharge from the hospital. The primary focus during this phase is awareness of loss and burn related changes, often major, in the patient's life. Dysphoric symptoms again include eating and sleep disturbances particularly nightmares, withdrawal from peer interactions, sad expression, an inability to enjoy anything and often tearfulness.

Case II: Intermediate Phase

The case of Thomas is an excellent example of a severely burned child at this level of treatment.

Thomas is a six-year-old boy who sustained partial and full thickness flame burns over 95% of his total body surface area. A younger sister was killed in the fire which occurred as the result of gasoline fumes igniting in his home.

During a long precarious acute stage, Thomas learned of his sister's death. He was told by his parents that "she went to heaven." He expressed some grief over this and suddenly stopped speaking about it.

As he began to improve steadily, he was transferred to the reconstructive ward. Thomas was a very serious and quiet child. He would eat only after much coaxing and cajoling. He refused to "play" but very much enjoyed being held and having stories read to him. When reading a Christmas story, "The Littlest Angel" he suddenly began to cry saying he didn't want to "hear anymore about that story." The reason for this uncharacteristically emotional outburst was because the boy in the story "went to heaven just like his sister." Thomas wept freely for some time and again that evening. Significantly he stated that he would not "be going to heaven for a long time until he was old." He had realized that he would survive the ordeal, and he could begin to grieve his sister's death.

The next day Thomas began to interact minimally with the other children in the playroom. He spoke more and more expressively. At this time, Thomas was wearing a face mask to put pressure on and flatten his facial scars. This made judging his facial expression impossible and made it difficult for staff and other children to be as spontaneously responsive to him as they might otherwise have been. Because of this problem, Thomas was allowed to remove his mask for several brief periods every day. Rapid social gains were noticed after this modification was instituted.

Thomas formed a particularly close relationship with his physical therapist who spent consistent time with him participating in game playing as well as painful physical therapy exercises. It was during a physical therapy session that Thomas first laughed, the first time he was able to stand and walk alone. A source of real enjoyment and pride were his new sneakers which were "just like everyone else's."

This case is an excellent example of a young boy who exhibited dysphoric affect when faced with a devastating burn, the loss of his sister and his temporary loss of mobility. He began to accept the reality of his situation and began to build upon it, wishing to be "just like everyone else."

The final stage of burn care, the rehabilitative, begins upon discharge from the hospital and continues for an indefinite period, until the child has successfully adapted to his environment. During this phase patients are often hospitalized for multiple reconstructive procedures. Children upon readmission sometimes remember the pain and unpleasantness associated with prior hospitalizations and become quite sad. They may exhibit this dysphoria in a forthright manner or by regressing to an earlier developmental level, i.e., bedwetting. The process of remembering their past experiences may trigger nightmares about these experiences.

We hear sad stories from children in the rehabilitative stage about how others have teased and isolated them as a result of their disfigurement. The following is an illustration of a young child in the rehabilitative phase.

Case III: Rehabilitative Phase

Beth is a five-year-old girl who sustained 55% total body surface area burns to her head, face, hands and chest. She was burned in a housefire. All three of her siblings were killed in the fire. Beth lost all of her fingers save her right thumb.

During her third reconstructive admission, approximately one and a half years after she was burned, Beth began to wet the bed nightly. She also slept fitfully and spoke about nightmares in which "monsters were trying to hurt her." Much of her time was spent playing alone. She cried frequently and verbalized how sad it was to be away from her mother.

When asked how things were at home Beth insisted all was well. However, in play therapy she presented another picture. Using a toy telephone, she called her "friend" at home, a boy about her age, and wept, pleading him not to call her funny names. These conversations continued for a week. Beth used them to reason with her little friend and stopped "calling" him when she knew he would like her because she enjoyed many of the same games and because she liked his jokes too.

Beth then initiated puppet play. Early during this phase she requested help constructing paper teeth for one of the puppets. Upon completion of the teeth she inserted them in the mouth of the puppet and proceeded to bite the hands of another puppet (a girl puppet with long blond hair not unlike her own) saying, "You don't need fingers, you really don't need them. I don't have them and I do good." After three or four minutes of this, Beth threw the puppets down and began to cry saying she missed her mother, and wanted to go home. When it was suggested that she might like to call her mother on the telephone, she perked up and agreed. She did speak with her mother, and arrangements were made for regular phone calls home. This cheered Beth immensely.

Beth designated a quilt found in the playroom as "the magic blanket," saying, "When you sit on this you can say anything and nothing will happen." She availed herself of this opportunity to express how sad and angry she was that her doctors had fixed her nose instead of her chin during this admission. This illustrates a dysphoric reaction often seen in young children who have, or feel that they have lost control over what is happening to their bodies. Shortly, Beth confronted her doctor about this. He explained to her in great detail why it was so important to fix her nose first. Children often use play as a means of working through their concerns around surgical issues. Frequently they do this by assuming the role of the doctor.

Prior to her discharge, Beth expressed very open and direct concerns about other children at home never wanting to play with her, and how unhappy it made her. Consultation with mother revealed that she had a tendency to over-protect Beth and isolate from experiences with a peer group so that she would not be teased. Realizing that this had become a problem for Beth, she expressed a willingness to provide her with more opportunities for peer group play activities.

Upon discharge, this plan was carried out with the support of the social worker and was successful. It provided Beth with a better social basis from which to enter school (Cahners, 1979; Cahners, Dumont, McLoughlin, & O'Connor, 1975).

This case points out how children who have returned to their home, school, etc., can make use of hospitalization to work through some of their sadness about their burn injury.

CONCLUSIONS

The management of dysphoria in severely burned young children is a team effort. During the acute phase we collaborate closely with pediatricians, surgeons and nurses, offering support to them as well as to the child and family. In the intermediate stage, we increase the scope of our activity to include recreation therapists, physical therapists and our school teacher. Throughout the rehabilitative process we have become involved with those in the community who are working with the child and his family. These professionals all play an important role in the quality of the child's life during hospitalization, and in the development of lifelong attitudes toward his burn injury.

If there is one message we would like to communicate, it is one of hope. To our constant amazement most of the severely burned children with whom we work cope remarkably well with the devasting consequences of their burns.

These children return to their homes, enter public school programs, join cub scouts, etc. Given a supportive family, they are able to work through the day-to-day problems that inevitably arise. The severely burned child generally does not exhibit chronic dysphoric symptomatology.

There are many questions as yet unanswered. We do not know how the children whose cases we shared with you will cope during adolescence or with the demands of adulthood. We are pleased to report that they seem to be functioning well now, and that we believe them to be quite representative of our younger population (Stoddard, 1981a). Only time and controlled research studies will bear out our clinical observations.

One thing appears likely. If we as professionals who work with these children and their families provide enough support, they follow the self-fulfilling prophecy. If they believe that they can adapt successfully to society, many of them can overcome the sadness, grief, withdrawal, and isolation experienced as a result of their burn trauma and return to a high level of psycho-social functioning in a relatively short period of time during their younger years.

REFERENCES

Antoon, A. Y., Volpe, J. J., Crawford, J. D. Burn encephalopathy in children. *Pediatrics,* 1972, *50*(4).

Bernstein, N. R. *The Emotional Care of the Facially Burned and Disfigured.* Boston: Little Brown and Co., 1976.

Branstetter, E. Separation anxiety and hospitalized children: Comparison from mothering. Doctoral dissertation in the Division of Social Sciences, University of Chicago, Chicago, 1969.

Cahners, S. S. A strong hospital-school liaison: A necessity for good rehabilitation planning for disfigured children. *Scandinavian Journal of Plastic and Reconstructive Surgery,* 1979, *13*:167-168.

Cahners, S. S., Dumont, J. McLoughlin, E., O'Connor, M. The burned child's return to school. Unpublished manuscript, 1975.

Diagnostic and statistical manual of mental disorders, third edition. Washington, D.C.: American Psychiatric Association, 1980.

Herrin, J. T., & Crawford, J. D. The seriously burned child. In Smith (Ed.), The critically ill child: Diagnosis and management. Philadelphia: W. B. Saunders, 1972.

Murray, G. G. Confusion, delirium and dementia. In T. P. Hackett & N. H. Cassem (Eds.), *Massachusetts General Hospital handbook of general hospital psychiatry.* St. Louis: C. V. Mosby Co., 1978.

Stoddard, F. J. Body image development in the burned child. Unpublished manuscript, 1980.

Stoddard, F. J. Coping with pain: Treatment of burned children from infancy to adolescence. *American Journal of Psychiatry,* 1981.

Stoddard, F. J. Here's Looking at You, Kid, a film review. *Community Mental Health Journal,* 1981, *17*(2).

Depression in Children
with Speech, Language,
and Learning Disorders

Dennis P. Cantwell MD
Lorian Baker, PhD

ABSTRACT. This paper reports on the prevalence of affective disorders in a sample of children presenting to a community clinic for speech or language evaluation. It was found that, among 600 children studied, 4% had some type of affective disorder, according to DSM-III diagnostic criteria. The children with affective disorders were generally not typical of the children presenting for speech and language evaluation: they tended to be older on the average, to have more psychiatric disorders, and to have more learning disorders than the "typical" child presenting for speech/language evaluation. The relationships between affective disorders, learning disorders, and speech/language disorders are discussed.

Children with handicaps of all types are known to be at risk for the development of psychiatric disorders. These include: intellectually retarded children, physically handicapped children, and brain damaged children. Two other handicaps that may predispose children to psychiatric problems are handicaps in communication (speech and language) and handicaps in learning. Rutter's review (1974) of the psychiatric literature found a strong association between the presence of learning disorders in childhood and various types of psychiatric problems. Our review (Cantwell and Baker, 1977) of the literature on children with communication disorders suggested that these children may have higher prevalence rates for psychiatric disorders than do children in the general population. Since language is a uniquely human quality, it is therefore not unex-

Dr. Cantwell is Joseph Campbell Professor of Child Psychiatry, and Dr. Baker is a Research Linguist. This work was supported by NIMH Grant MH27919. Drs. Cantwell and Baker are located at the University of California at Los Angeles, Neuropsychiatric Institute, 760 Westwood Plaza, Los Angeles, CA 90024.

51

pected that a disorder in language development might have far-reaching consequences for other areas of early childhood development. In fact, systematic research has suggested that language is uniquely and intrinsically related to the development of the child's thought, play activities, social and emotional development and learning (Baker and Cantwell, in press).

For the past several years, the present authors have been involved in a large-scale study examining psychiatric disorder in a sample of children with communication disorders. The present paper will report on some of the findings from that study. In particular, the prevalence and types of affective disorders occurring in children with speech and language disorder will be examined, and the interrelationships between speech and language disorder will be examined, and the interrelationships between speech and language disorder, learning disorders, and affective disorders will be discussed.

Methods

The methodology of this study has been described in detail elsewhere (Cantwell et al., 1979; 1980). Briefly, we selected for study children presenting for speech and language evaluation at a community speech and hearing clinic in the greater Los Angeles area. The clinic chosen draws its patients from a population area of over one million inhabitants and serves a wide range of socioeconomic classes. All children between the ages of 2 and 16 years presenting to this clinic for speech and language evaluation were asked to participate in the study. Children presenting to the clinic for pure audiologic evaluations were excluded from participation. The refusal rate for participation in the study was less than 3%.

In addition to the informal speech evaluation done by the speech clinic staff, each child received a detailed linguistic evaluation by a psycholinguist (LB) which included both formal tests (the Goldman-Fristoe Test of Articulation, the Illinois Test of Psycholinguistic Abilities, the Peabody Picture Vocabulary Test, the Carrow Test of Auditory Comprehension of Language), and linguistic analysis of a free-speech sample.

A detailed psychiatric evaluation was also done on each child. The evaluation consisted of a semi-structured psychiatric interview with the parents about the child, a semi-structured interview with the child, and the use of parent and teacher behavior rating scales. The parent and teacher rating scales were slightly modified from those developed by Rutter, Tizard, and Whitmore (1970) and Connors (1970). A psychiatric diagnosis was made based on all the information obtained in the interview with the parent, the interview with the child, and the parent and teacher rating scales.

The general definition of a psychiatric disorder in this study is modified from that listed in the introduction to the Diagnostic and Statistical Manual for Mental Disorders (DSM-III) (APA, 1980). A child was considered to have a psychiatric disorder if he demonstrated a disorder of behavior, emotions, cognition, or relationships, which was sufficiently prolonged and/or sufficiently severe to cause distress, disability, or disadvantage to the child and/or disturbance in his or her environment. If a psychiatric disorder was determined to be present, a specific diagnosis was made based on the criteria described in DSM-III.

Intellectual ability and academic achievement were assessed using the Wechsler Intelligence Scale for Children or the Wechsler Pre-School and Primary Scale of Intelligence (depending on the child's age), the Peabody Vocabulary Test, the Wide-Range Achievement Test, and the Gray Oral Reading Test. In addition, information was provided by means of questionnaires completed by the children's teachers. These questionnaires included information on what problems the child had at the time, if any; how long the teacher had known the child; the results of any recent standardized intelligence academic achievement test; how well the child was achieving in various school subjects; whether a special placement was necessary in school; whether academic help or referral to a mental health specialist was required; and an overall rating of the child's problem. The teacher was also asked to rate the severity of the child's problem in four specific areas on a four-point scale: behavior, academic achievement, group participation, and attitude towards authority.

The diagnosis of learning ability or disability was made according to DSM-III operational diagnostic criteria and using data from the intelligence testing, the academic testing, and the school teachers' questionnaires.

Results

Children Studied: Six hundred children between the ages of two and sixteen years were evaluated in this study. Sixty-nine percent of these children were males, and the mean age of the group was 5 years, 10 months.

Approximately one-half of the 600 children were found to have some diagnosable psychiatric disorder according to DSM-III diagnostic criteria for axis 1. A small percentage of the children were found to have more than one psychiatric axis 1 disorder.

The most common major grouping of psychiatric disorders were overt behavior disorders, which affected 26% of the sample. Emotional disorders were nearly as common, affecting 19% of the sample. The single most common diagnosis was attention deficit disorder with hyperactivity, which affected 17% of the children.

Thirty-four percent of the children in the sample were diagnosed as having a pure speech disorder (that is, a disorder of articulation, fluency or voice, but with language comprehension, expression, and processing within normal limits). Eight percent of the 600 children were found to have a pure language disorder (a disorder involving the comprehension, or expression or processing of grammar, vocabulary or syntax, with speech articulation, fluency and voicing within normal limits). The majority of the children in the sample (58%) had a disorder involving both speech and language.

Learning disorders were found in 7% of the children. Considering that the majority of the children in the study were in the preschool age range, this number is surprisingly large. Of the learning disabilities identified, the most frequently occurring type was mixed specific learning disorder, which affected 26 children (or 4% of the sample). Specific reading disorder was the second most commonly occurring disorder, affecting 13 children (or 2% of the sample).

Table I presents the data on the 600 children studied, as well as on the subgroups of children with learning disorders and affective disorders.

Children with Affective Disorders. Affective disorders were found in a total of 23 children (or 4% of the sample). The data presented in Table 1 reveals some interesting findings regarding the children who had an affective disorder diagnosis. First, although the sex distribution (16 males and 7 females) is the same sex distribution as in the total sample, the age distribution of the depressed group is not. These children are considerably older with a mean age of 11 years. Also, the depressed children were much more likely to have a pure language disorder. Only 45 of the entire population of 600 children had a pure language disorder and 9 of them are in the group of 23 who had a major affective disorder diagnosis. Likewise, the children with affective disorder are more likely to have another Axis

Table 1: Children Studied

	Whole Sample of Speech and Language Disordered Children	Affective Disorders Subgroup	Learning Disorders Subgroup
Number of Children	600	23*	42*
Age (Range and Mean)	2 yrs, 0 mos - 15 yrs, 11 mos; 5 yrs, 10 mos	6 yrs, 6 mos - 15 yrs, 11 mos; 11 yrs, 0 mos	4 yrs, 6 mos - 15 yrs, 11 mos; 9 yrs, 10 mos
Sex (% Male)	69%	70%	64%
Verbal I.Q. (Range and Mean)	20-150; 95.8	68-144; 100.0	55-146; 93.9
Performance I.Q. (Range and Mean)	20-150; 105.1	76-155; 111.0	73-152; 98.0
Psychiatric Diagnoses:			
None	n=298 (49.7%)	n=0 (0)	n=11 (26%)
One	n=272 (45%)	n=12 (52%)	n=7 (17%)
More than one	n=30 (5%)	n=11 (48%)	n=24 (57%)
Linguistic Diagnoses:			
Pure Speech Disorder	n=203 (34%)	n=6 (26%)	n=6 (14%)
Speech & Language Disorder	n=352 (58%)	n=8 (35%)	n=26 (62%)
Pure Language Disorder	n=45 (8%)	n=9 (39%)	n=10 (24%)
Learning Disorders:			
None	n=558 (93%)	n=15 (65%)	n=0
Specific Arithmetic	n=1 (<1%)	n=0 (0)	n=1 (2%)
Specific Reading	n=13 (2%)	n=1 (4%)	n=13 (31%)
Mixed	n=26 (4%)	n=7 (31%)	n=26 (62%)
Atypical	n=2 (<1%)	n=0 (0)	n=2 (5%)

* Note: There is an overlap between the learning disordered and affective disordered groups with seven cases having both disorders.

55

I diagnosis. Only 30 of the entire population of 600 children had more than one Axis I psychiatric diagnosis. However, 11 of the 23 children with an affective disorder diagnosis had another Axis I diagnosis. Attention deficit disorder, the most common Axis I diagnosis found in the sample of 600 children, was present in 9 of these 11 children. Finally, one-third of the children with an affective disorder diagnosis had some specific learning disorder diagnosable using DSM-III criteria. This is considerably more than the 7% of children in the total sample who had learning disabilities.

Children with Learning Disorders: The learning disordered subgroup of communication impaired children consisted of 42 children who were different in several ways from the overall sample of children with communication disorders. First, the learning disordered children tended to be older than the overall sample. Performance intelligence scores were slightly lower on the average in the learning disabled group, although none of the learning disabled children tested in the mentally retarded range. The prevalence of psychiatric disorders was higher in the learning disabled subgroup than in the overall sample. A greater proportion of children in the learning disabled group had pure language disorders, and a smaller proportion had pure speech disorders than in the overall sample.

It is of interest to note that of the 42 children in the learning disorders subgroup, 7 were also in the affective disorders subgroup. This means that 17% of the learning disordered communication impaired children suffered from an affective disorder. The learning disabled group as a whole resembled the affective disordered group in a number of ways: Both of these subgroups were older on the average than the overall sample, both tended to have more psychiatric disorders than the overall sample, and both tended to have fewer pure speech disorders than the overall sample. However, the learning disabled group was different from the affective disordered subgroup in several ways: The learning disordered group tended to be younger, to have lower verbal intelligence levels, to have fewer psychiatric disorders, and to have more combined speech and language disorders than the affective disorders group.

Types of Affective Disorders Found. Table 2 gives a breakdown of those who met diagnostic criteria for one of the DSM-III affective disorders, including major depression, single episode dysthymic disorder, cyclothymic disorder, and bipolar disorder, manic. In addition to the 23 children with true affective disorder, there were also 2 children with a diagnosis of adjustment disorder with depressed

Table 2: Children with Affective Disorder

	Major Depression Single Episode	Dysthymic Disorder	Cyclothymic Disorder	Bipolar Disorder
Number of Cases	10	5	7	1
Age Range and Mean	6 yrs 6 mos - 11 yrs 1 mo 8 yrs 6 mos	8 yrs 11 mos - 15 yrs 8 mos 13 yrs 1 mo	8 yrs 6 mo - 15 yrs 11 mos 12 yrs 6 mos	15 yrs 5 mos
Sex (% Males)	90%	40%	71%	0
Linguistic Diagnoses:				
Pure Speech Disorder	n=3 (30%)	n=1 (20%)	n=2 (29%)	0
Speech and Language Disorder	n=3 (30%)	n=3 (60%)	n=2 (29%)	n=1 (100%)
Pure Language Disorder	n=6 (40%)	n=1 (20%)	n=3 (42%)	0
Verbal I.Q. (Range and Mean)	87-121 105.2	75-144 100.8	68-135 93.0	93
Performance I.Q. (Range and Mean)	83-155 116.4	80-122 103.0	76-143 113.6	80
Axis I Syndromes:				
No Other Disorders	n=4 (40%)	n=3 (60%)	n=4 (57%)	n=1 (100%)
Attention Deficit Disorder	n=6 (60%)	n=1 (20%)	n=2 (29%)	0
Parent-Child Problem	0	n=1 (20%)	n=1 (14%)	0
Axis II Disorders:				
No Disorders	n=3 (30%)	n=3 (60%)	n=2 (29%)	0
Encopresis/Enuresis	n=4 (40%)	n=0	n=1 (14%)	0
Coordination Disorder	n=1 (10%)	n=0	n=0	0
Specific Reading Disorder	n=1 (10%)	n=2 (40%)	n=0	0
Mixed Specific Learning Disorder	n=1 (10%)	0	n=3 (86%)	n=1 (100%)

mood. Thus, 25 children had a diagnosis with primary affective symptomatology.

Although the numbers of children suffering from affective disorders are too small for statistical comparison across specific diagnoses, it appears that the children with single episode major depressions are younger, more predominantly males, more frequently suffering from a secondary Axis I psychiatric disorder, and more frequently developmentally disordered than are the children with other types of affective disorders.

Discussion

Our study revealed that 23 of 600 children referred for early speech and language delay to a community speech and hearing clinic met DSM-III criteria for some affective diagnosis. These children tended to be older than the average child who came to the clinic, were more likely to have a pure language disorder, another Axis I psychiatric diagnosis in addition to their affective disorder diagnosis, and a specific learning disorder.

It is noteworthy that Kashani (personal communication) in a study of 100 children referred to a community mental health center in Columbia, Missouri, found that one-half of all children who were given an affective disorder diagnosis also had a developmental language disorder. This is an intriguing association which we have not seen mentioned before.

We have previously discussed (Cantwell and Baker, 1977) the hypothesized mechanisms by which a speech and language disorder may be associated with a psychiatric disorder. These include the fact that they may both have possible common antecedents such as intellectual retardation, deafness, brain damage, family factors, social class, and psychosocial stressors occurring in the child's life. Our previous analyses (Cantwell et al., 1979; 1980) of early data from this study showed that none of these factors played a strong role in the etiology of the psychiatric disorder. Children with a language disorder and a speech and language disorder were much more likely to have a psychiatric disorder than children with a pure speech disorder.

We also found a strong correlation between the presence of academic failure and the presence of a psychiatric disorder. While in those without academic failure and those with academic failure the most common diagnosis is attention deficit disorder with hyperactivity, there are a number of those children who also have an affective disorder. Many of those without an affective disorder did have affective symptomatology as a primary part of their psychopathology.

In summary, it does seem clear that children with early speech and language delay are at risk for the development of psychiatric disorder and that affective symptomatology may predominate in some of these children. The presence of affective disorders in speech and language disordered children appears to be limited to a specific subset of communication impaired children who tend to be older, more frequently learning disabled, and less frequently speech impaired, than the children typically presenting to a speech clinic. The presence of affective disorder in these children would be likely to interfere with their social, emotional, and academic functioning which are already compromised by their speech and language delay. We believe it is important that these children are identified in schools or speech clinics and are given comprehensive treatment.

REFERENCES

American Psychiatric Association. *Diagnostic and statistical manual of mental disorders* (3rd ed.). Washington, D.C.: The American Psychiatric Association, 1980.

Baker, L., & Cantwell, D. P. Language acquisition, cognitive development, and emotional disorder in childhood. In K. Nelson (Ed.), *Children's language* (Vol. 3). New York: Gardner Press, Inc., in press.

Cantwell, D. P., & Baker, L. Psychiatric disorder in children with speech and language retardation: A critical review. *Archives of General Psychiatry*, 1977, *34*, 583-591.

Cantwell, D. P., Baker, L., & Mattison, R. Factors associated with the development of psychiatric disorder in children with speech and language retardation. *Archives of General Psychiatry*, 1980, *37*, 423-426.

Cantwell, D. P., Baker, L., & Mattison, R. The prevalence of psychiatric disorder in children with speech and language disorder: An epidemiological study. *Journal of the American Academy of Child Psychiatry*, 1979, *18*, 450-461.

Conners, C. K. Rating scales for use in drug studies with children. *Psychopharmacology Bulletin*. Rockville, Maryland: Department of Health, Education and Welfare (Early Clinical Drug Evaluation Unit), 1970.

Rutter, M. Emotional disorders and educational underachievement. *Archives of General Psychiatry*, 1974, *49*, 249-256.

Rutter, M., Tizard, J., & Whitmore, K. (Eds.) *Education, health, and behavior.* London: Longmans & Green, 1970.

TREATMENT

The Causes and Treatment of Depression in Young Children

Brian J. McConville, MB, ChB, FRCP(C)

ABSTRACT. Symptoms of sadness and misery occur frequently in children, but do not always cause frank depressive symptoms, or minor or major childhood affective disorders. This paper indicates some studies suggesting that although most children adapt quickly, sustained depression and cumulative losses cause more severe conditions. In younger children, affectual themes predominate, but with older children with more sustained losses there is an evolution into negative self-esteem symptoms which are difficult to reverse with psychotherapy or pharmacotherapy. The classical guilt depression are uncommon, but respond well to pharmacotherapy. Early identification and treatment of childhood depressive disorders is essential.

Life events causing stress, loss and deprivation in young children give rise to sadness and misery, or more frank depressive symptoms which may eventually be associated with minor or major affective disorders. Alternatively, children's responses may diminish with time, with consequent resolution, or even increased adaptation. Lois Murphy (1962) commented on the complex adaptational maneuvers made by quite young children to stress, and despite the initial concern of Bowlby (1952) about the effects of maternal deprivation, Tizard (1975), and Rutter (1971,1972) have shown that these effects

Brian J. McConville is Professor of Psychiatry, Queen's University, Kingston, Ontario.

are not inevitable. Poznanski et al. (1976) state that chronic and sustained privation appears to be more important than single traumatic deprivation in determining chronic conditions. Moreover, deprivation experiences can be ameliorated following appropriate care, or worsened by chronic family or social problems.

Initially, Wolfenstein (1966) suggested that "true" mourning and depression were impossible for a child until adolescence, although Bowlby (1960) felt that no qualitative difference existed between child and adult mourning-depressive responses. Freud (1960), Schur (1960), and Spitz (1960) took an intermediate view that a child's mourning-depressive response was a function of age and developmental stage and an active debate took place. Current clinical concerns are more with the phenomenology of different depressive responses in children at varying ages and developmental stages, rather than whether phenomena are consistent or not with a particular theory.

A further question is whether children's depressive responses differ with age, developmental stage, and previous experience. This paper describes some studies of particular life events giving rise to sustained depressive symptoms in young children, including the transformation into the minor or major affective disorders of childhood described by Puig-Antich (1980), Carlson and Cantwell (1979), and Petti (1978).

Children's Depressive Responses to Acute and Severe Loss

One area of loss studied is that of children's reaction to death, as a dramatic and often unexpected event providing a finite area for observation. A particularly poignant example is that of children facing their own terminal illness. In such children, age variations clearly occur. Schowalter (1970) wrote that children under three were preoccupied with separation from a mothering or caring person, but from three to six the child often saw his death as a retribution for bad thoughts and actions. Children aged six to nine conceptualized and feared death as an external force which had stopped the lives of others, and might stop theirs. After age ten the irreversibility and permanence of death were better internalized and altruistic concern for others began to appear.

These concepts appear based on the child's cognitive concepts of death at various ages, consistent with the work of Nagy (1965). However, Gartley and Bernasconi (1967) found that the stages were not invariant; younger children's belief that death was personified and reversible was probably modifiable by religious experience.

The children described above had different physical illnesses, and also different family backgrounds. In contrast, some years ago we had the chance to study a group of children in a residential setting following the dramatic death of two key caring people. The director and co-director both died in a fire in the house where they lived (McConville et al., 1976).

Following this tragic event all children were administered a standard interview within two weeks after the fire, with a follow-up interview after ten to twelve weeks. The recorded interviews were rated by two child psychiatrists, with satisfactory reliability on given items. Significant differences were found between the younger (five to eight) and the older (nine to twelve) children. Younger children showed simpler coping mechanisms such as comments on their own centrality in events related to the fire, regression to earlier immature patterns, denial, animistic fantasies and preoccupations with the dead, and simple restitutive dreams that the dead people were still alive. Older children showed more concern for others, and more general adaptation. However, by the time of the second interview most of the significant differences between younger and older children had disappeared, as the younger children appeared to have adapted reasonably well. Intelligence, number of placements, and time spent at the treatment setting did not correlate significantly with responses to loss or general adaptation of the child either at the first or second interview, so that the effect of these factors could not be clearly established.

The therapy provided was to give each child constant support, explanation and exploration of the child's feelings about the deaths, utilizing a particular child care worker for each child. The children's mourning depressive responses subsided, but sporadic episodes of extreme grief happened often, especially in the younger children. Consistent with the findings of Cytryn and McKnew (1972) and Carlson and Cantwell (1979), frank depression was not always present, but underlying depressive fantasies were common. Real or symbolic loss often caused underlying depression to become more evident. For example, for one girl, the subsequent loss of a loved teacher who went off to have her baby rather prematurely occasioned an outburst of intense anger and resentment, along with concerns that she too might die.

This study gave some support for the notion of age differences in mourning-depressive themes, but also showed that adaptation could occur even in a severely deprived group of children, at least at a superficial level. A group of normal children whose teacher had died were studied at the same time; they showed similar depressive themes, but appeared to get over the event more quickly. Perhaps then, children who had had cumulative earlier experience of severe loss and deprivation are affected more deeply than those who had only experienced ordinary life crises. This concept is in part consistent with the study of Kashani et al. (1981), where hospitalized children aged 7 to 12 had significantly more dysphoric moods and full depressions on the B.I.D. (Petti, 1978) and DSM-III (APA, 1970) criteria, than a group of non-hospitalized children from the general population.

In summary there is considerable evidence that children respond clearly to acute stress, loss and deprivation, but there are also indications that their responses are often not sustained, and that supporting social and family structures can modify these age-related responses.

Children's Depressive Responses to More Chronic Stress and Loss

Following this initial study of depressive responses to a common loss, we investigated more severe depressive symptoms in a group of children hospitalized for psychiatric care. This group had a variety of organic/cognitive, social/behavioral and affectual/intrapsychic primary symptoms. A primary symptom of depression was present in 51 percent, and 6 percent had a full diagnosis of affective disorder, consonant with overall figures described for similar groups by Carlson and Cantwell (1979), Petti (1978), and Weinberg (1973). Fifteen verbally expressed depressive themes that were observed most frequently and these fell into three groups. Five items in the first group related to expressed sadness, helplessness, loneliness, loss and a general feeling of being bad; these were the affectual depression sub-group (D-1). The second group of five items related to negative self-esteem (D-2), with expressed concerns of being no-good or punk, of being unable to help or do things for others, and of being unliked, along with long-term expectations of being used or exploited, and an estimate that the situation would not change. A third group included feelings of being wicked, hated and justly punished, with wishes to kill oneself, or to be dead, associated with restitutive fantasies. These constituted the guilt depression for sub-type (D-3). Each item was noted in terms of frequency and intensity of reference in the first six weeks of the assessment period, and two child psychiatrists also rated the child on a structured interview, with adequate reliability in two independent settings. It was found that affectual (D-1) items were significantly more common than negative self-esteem items in younger children (Freud, 1960; Kashani, 1980), while negative self-esteem items became more common than affectual at age 8-12 and became steadily more common with increasing age. The guilt (D-3) items began from age 10 and always followed extreme traumatic events such as the loss of one's brother by sudden death. The three sub-groups were combined to give a total depression score, which also increased with age. Hence the different sub-types were not independent of each other, but represented the interplay of affectual and cognitive factors in children at different ages (McConville et al., 1972).

Recent traumatic loss preceded the guilt depressions but were uncommon in the group overall, suggesting that acute losses were usually well handled. In a further study of this group (McConville et al., 1976) 73 inpatients with moderate to severe depression scores were identified. Boys were more common than girls, but the ratio was similar to that seen for other disorders within the unit. Seventy percent of the children had significant bereavement or loss of parents or siblings, and usually such losses had occurred cumulatively over time. Fifty-one percent of the group had suffered significant rejection by their parents or parent figures over the previous three years, and significant parental depression had occurred in 63% of parents, with the majority occurring in mothers.

The overall multidisciplinary therapy approaches for this group were complex, but resemble those described by Petti et al. (1980) in their evaluation and multimodality treatment of a depressed prepubertal girl.

Individual psychotherapy showed differences between the clinical sub-types, largely because of the way in which the child related to the therapist. In younger children with predominantly affectual depressions, the initial relationship was intense and based on an early parent/child model stressing body contact, "being with" and structured nurturance. Initially the child's expressed sadness and wishes to die decreased, and he became more spontaneously affectionate. But in the middle phase of therapy themes of being harmed or killed by the therapist or by frightening fantasy figures often emerged. In a final phase the child was able to accept affection, with increased self-esteem and decreased demandingness.

In contrast, older children with predominantly negative self-esteem often had a basic mistrust of the therapist, and goals had to be set concretely in terms of what it was worth to the child to form relationships. Long-term arrangements for nurturance needed to be spelled out clearly and the child began slowly to trust, with frequent periods of angry rejection where he maintained that he did not need or wish for help. Later more clinging behavior often occurred, with some internalization of other's standards and associated guilt for rejecting behavior.

The uncommon predominantly guilt depressions had a high risk of suicide, often with related auditory hallucinations. The therapist was initially supportive but also limit setting towards the self-destructive impulses, and with later reality oriented planning. Those with mixed affectual and negative self-esteem depressions showed combinations of the first two responses to therapy.

In pharmacotherapy for the depressed children, the guilt depression sub-type responded promptly to use of tricyclic antidepressants, but the other sub-types responded less clearly. It would seem that responses to antidepressants may vary with severity and sub-type of the depressive disorder, consistent with the studies of Lucas et al. (1965), Weinberg et al. (1973), Puig-Antich et al. (1980) and Petti et al. (1980) on children with pre-pubertal major depressive disorders.

The overall results in our study were that the guilt depressions responded best to drug and psychotherapy treatment, judged by changes in the total depression scores at discharge and follow-up, and by time spent in treatment. Affectual depressions and the mixed D-1 and D-2 sub-type depressions responded less well, and the negative self-esteem depressions responded worst on the above criteria. All differences were significant.

Current studies are underway to indicate how these depressive items fit into more general classifications of depression such as the B.I.D. and the DSM-III, while retaining questions regarding differences in age, sex and prior experience as criteria to be investigated in childhood depression.

In summary, our studies have suggested that there may be a progression of responses, especially in younger children, from early affectual responses involving sadness, grief and a need for nurturing persons into a colder and non-accepting pattern of depressive responses characterized by self-hatred, and by change in the child's cognitive perception. Lewis & Lewis (1979) recently suggested following Mandell (1976), that sustained monoamine transmitter depletion in children might follow chronic deprivation experiences. Perhaps these ideas could inter-relate.

Children have considerable plasticity to stress, especially in the context of a supportive family and social matrix. But prolonged deprivation and loss in a non-caring environment, and especially where parenting figures are diffuse, negative or unknown, seems to provide for a long-term deleterious effect. Those with frank major affective disorders may respond well to pharmacotherapy, although a recent controlled study of imipramine by Puig-Antich (1980), casts doubt on this. But many depressed children do not clearly fit into this category, and may have rather debilitating and long-term depressive symptoms or minor affective disorders. Especially for children with chronic negative self-esteem, the results of either drug therapy or psychotherapy often seem to be poor, and the possibility of uncared for children being unable to care for others in due course is high. There is therefore a strong need for early intervention in children showing depressive symptoms, with caring therapists allowing for mourning and restructuring before more permanent changes occur.

REFERENCES

American Psychiatric Association. Diagnostic and Statistical Manual (III). Washington, D.C., 1970.

Bowlby, J. Grief and mourning in infancy and early childhood. In *The Psychoanalytic Study of the Child*. New York: International Universities Press, 1960, *15*, 9-52.

Bowlby, J. *Maternal Care and Mental Health*. Geneva: World Health Organization, 1952.

Carlson, G. and Cantwell, D. A survey of depressive symptoms in a child and adolescent psychiatric population. *Journal of the American Academy of Child Psychiatry*, 1979, *18*, 587-599.

Cytryn, L. and McKnew, D. Proposed classification of childhood depressions. *American Journal of Psychiatry*, 1972, *129*, 149-155.

Freud, A. Discussion of Dr. John Bowlby's paper. In *The Psychoanalytic Study of the Child*. New York: International Universities Press, 1960, *15*, 53-62.

Gartley, W. and Bernasconi, M. The concept of death in children. *Journal of Genetic Psychology*, 1967, *110*, 71-85.

Kashani, J., Barbero, G., & Bolander, F. Depression in hospitalized pediatric patients. *Journal of the American Academy of Child Psychiatry*, 1981, *20*, 123-134.

Lewis, M. and Lewis D. A psycho-biological view of childhood depression. In A. French (Ed.), *Clinical Approaches to Childhood Depression*. New York: Human Sciences Press, 1979.

Lucas, A., Locket, H. and Grimm, F. Amitriptyline in child depressions. *Diseases of the Nervous System*, 1965, *26*, 105-110.

Mandell, A. Neurobiological mechanism of adaptation in relation to models of psycho-biological development. In E. Schopler & R. Reichler (Eds.), *Psychopathology and Child Development*. New York: Plenum, 1976.

McConville, B. and Boag, L. Therapeutic approaches in childhood depression. Paper read at the American Academy of Child Psychiatry Meeting, Toronto, 1976.

McConville, B., Boag, L. and Purohit, A. Mourning depressive responses of children in residence following sudden death of parent figures. *Journal of the American Academy of Child Psychiatry,* 1972, *11,* 341-364.

McConville, B., Boag, L. and Purohit, A. Three types of childhood depression. *Canadian Psychiatric Association Journal,* 1973, *18,* 133-138.

Murphy, L. *The Widening World of Childhood.* New York: Basic Books, 1962.

Nagy, M. The child's view of death. In H. Feifel (Ed.), *The Meaning of Death.* New York: McGraw-Hill, 1965, 79-98.

Petti, T. Depression in hospitalized child psychiatry patients. *Journal of the American Academy of Child Psychiatry,* 1978, *17,* 49-59.

Petti, T., Bornstein, M., Delamater, A. and Conners, C. Evaluation and multimodality treatment of a depressed prepubertal girl. *Journal of the American Academy of Child Psychiatry,* 1980, *19,* 690-702.

Poznanski, E., Krahenbuhl, V. and Zrull, J. Childhood depression: A longitudinal perspective. *Journal of the American Academy of Child Psychiatry,* 1976, *15,* 491-501.

Puig-Antich, J. Affective disorders in childhood: A review and perspective. *Psychiatric Clinics of North America,* 1980, *3,* 403-424.

Puig-Antich, J., Blau, S., Marx, N. et. al. Prepubertal major depressive disorder: Pilot study. *Journal of the American Academy of Child Psychiatry,* 1978, *17,* 695-707.

Puig-Antich, J., Perel, J., Lupatkin, W. et al. Plasma levels of imipramine (IMI) and desmethylimipramine on clinical response to prepubertal major depressive disorder. *Journal of the American Academy of Child Psychiatry,* 1979, 616-627.

Rutter, M. *Maternal Deprivation Reassessed.* Harmondsworth, Penguin, 1972.

Rutter, M. Parent-child separation: Psychological effects on the children. *Journal of Child Psychology and Psychiatry,* 1971, *12,* 233-260.

Schowalter, J. The child's reaction to his own terminal illness. In B. Schoenberg (Ed.), *Loss and Grief: Psychological Management in Medical Practice,* New York: Columbia University Press, 1970, 51-69.

Schur, N. Discussion of Dr. John Bowlby's paper. In *The Psychoanalytic Study of the Child.* New York: International Universities Press, 1960, *15,* 63-84.

Spitz, R. Discussion of Dr. John Bowlby's paper. In *The Psychoanalytic Study of the Child.* New York: International Universities Press, 1960, *15,* 85-94.

Tizard, B. and Rees, J. The effect of early institutional rearing on the behaviour problems and affectional relationships of four-year-old children. *Journal of Child Psychology and Psychiatry,* 1975, *16,* 61-74.

Weinberg, W., Rutman, J., Sullivan, L. et al. Depression in children referred to an educational diagnostic centre: Diagnosis and treatment. *Journal of Pediatrics,* 1973, *83,* 1065-1072.

Wolfenstein, M. *How is mourning possible?* In *The Psycholanalytic Study of the Child.* New York: International Universities Press, 1966, *21,* 93-123.

Intervention and Prevention Strategies for Children with Depressed Mothers

John D. O'Brien, MD

Motherhood is a developmental process which requires changes on the mother's part as the child grows and his needs and personality change. Maternal depression disrupts the mutual activation and regulation that characterizes a healthy mother-child relationship. Preschool children of depressed mothers have a high incidence of behavioral disorders, difficulty in eating, difficulty in obtaining bladder control and a high accident rate. The first intervention strategy is to heighten awareness of front line care taking personnel to the prevalence and effects of the problem. Educational, environmental manipulation, psychopharmacological and psychotherapeutic means need to be used to intervene in and prevent the effects on both mother and child.

DEPRESSION IN MOTHERS

It has been only within the last ten years that sustained efforts have been made to investigate the effects of maternal depression on children at various stages in their development. Now that the effects are better understood, clinicians and researchers are beginning to explore prevention and treatment programs that can ameliorate this condition.

Definition

The word depression has various meanings and is used by many people to express a variety of emotional states ranging from disappointment to suicidal feelings. It is essential to have a clear definition for research purposes, for clear and meaningful communication

John D. O'Brien is Assistant Clinical Professor of Psychiatry, Cornell University-Medical Center, and Director of Child and Adolescent Psychiatry, St. Vincent's Hospital and Medical Center, 144 West 12th Street, New York, New York 10011.

among colleagues, and for clear and consistent communication with patients. Moreover, in efforts at primary and secondary prevention, families and their children must clearly understand depression and it is essential that the definition be stated in terms commensurate with their cognitive abilities. Depression can be a normal mood experienced by everybody or it can become abnormal when it persists over a period of time and adversely affects the everyday functioning of the person.

When the depressed mood persists over a period of time, the following symptoms are likely to occur: feelings of apathy, of helplessness, of hopelessness, and unworthiness; lack of pleasure; and problems in concentrating. Frequently, the depressed person alludes to the fact that "nothing seems to go right" or "I never seem to be able to please them." Along with these feelings, it is common to observe states of anxiety which are often expressed through bodily manifestations.

Accompanying these feelings, maybe there is a loss of appetite, the existence of sleep problems, irritability, and agitation. In severe depression, a person may become psychotic and be unable to recognize the reality of situations. Suicidal thoughts or actions may occur; often these thoughts have a passive quality to them like "why don't I just die."

Epidemiology

Epidemological studies have demonstrated the common occurrence of depression in mothers of young children. Brown (1975) found an overall prevalence of depression in women of 16%; in working class women with children under age six, a rate of 42% was found as compared to 25% in working class and 5% in middle class women. Moss and Plewis (1977) found 5% of the mothers with pre-school children to have had a moderate to severe "distress" over the previous year. Kendall (1976) showed a new episode rate for functional psychosis and depressive reactions to rise sharply in the first three months after delivery followed by a less dramatic but more sustained rise in the tenth to twenty-fourth month. Wolkind (1980) in a longitudinal study of primiparous women (women bearing their first child) found 10% of randomly selected mothers to be depressed throughout the first 3-4 years of the child's life.

IMPACT OF DEPRESSION ON MOTHERHOOD

The depression found in mothers of young children has a power-ful effect on marital and family life as well as the development and health of the children. It has been documented for some time that children of parents with chronic physical or psychiatric illnesses have more psychopathology and behavior problems than children of well parents (Anthony, 1969; Ekdahl, 1962; Orvaschel, 1981; Rut-ter, 1966). Welner (1977) found that children of mothers hospitalized for depression had a significantly higher incidence of depression than those of well mothers. Direct studies of children of bipolar manic depressives (Kestenbaum, 1981; McKnew, 1979; O'Connell, 1979) showed 40-55% of the children to be symptomatic and merit a psychiatric diagnosis. A high proportion were depressed and other symptomatology included psychosis, behavior disturbance and anx-iety attacks.

We can now look at how the symptoms effect the mother-child relationship and how this reverberates on the child. Motherhood is a developmental process which requires changes on the part of the mother as the child grows and his needs and personality change. Mothers need to adapt to this ever-changing organism so that future maturation of the child can take place. The effectiveness with which a mother resolves the issues at hand is dependent not only on her personality and her state of being but also on the manner in which the child presents her with his needs. Whenever a mother is unable to perceive correctly or respond congruently to the needs or inten-tions of the child there is a maladaptive resolution of the issue or issues confronting the dyad or family.

Weissman (1972) found depressed mothers to be significantly im-paired as mothers showed diminished emotional investment in the child, impaired communication, disaffection and increased hostility and resentment. This hostility is directly related to the degree of in-timacy and ranges from irritability and arguments to physical en-counters.

IMPACT ON CHILD'S DEVELOPMENTAL STAGES

There have been several schemata (Sanders, 1964; Weissman, 1972) used to conceptualize the needs of a child at a given develop-mental stage and the corresponding tasks required of the mother to meet those needs.

Infancy

In the newborn period, the mother needs to be able to meet the physical needs of the child, to establish mutuality between the child and herself, and to be able to separate her own needs from those of the child. Zax (1977), in studying the effects of maternal schizophrenia on children, used women with neurotic depression as one of the comparison groups. The research study revealed that children of depressed mothers become more symptomatic than children of schizophrenic or well mothers. The babies of depressed mothers have lower Apgar scores, low birth weights, and a higher incidence of fetal deaths. In the classic postpartum depression, mothers feel helpless and overwhelmed by the new child and the new role of motherhood.

For the mothers to protect themselves against these feelings and ultimately feeling of failure, they will withdraw from the caring of their infant because they feel they are "not good enough" or they become increasingly preoccupied with the infant in an over protective manner, e.g., frequently overfeeding the child or being fearful of holding or leaving the child. The child is affected the most and has the greatest of difficulties when the depressed mother directs her aggressive acts or hostile behavior directly at him or when the mother's anxiety or irritability results in restrictive caring or pathological neglect. This is especially true in postpartum psychoses where the mother may be unable to provide for the physical needs of the child and the father; other family members or outside people must be called in to substitute for the mother while she receives the appropriate treatment.

Preschool Age

As the child gets older, the mother must assist the child in separating from her and in seeing himself as a unique entity. It is well documented that this task is a great stress for some mothers; they need to keep the child in a helpless, dependent position. Likewise, it is common for women to have several children in a row "so I can always have a little one around." Behavioral problems are the most common difficulties found in preschool children of depressed mothers. The child is likely to have temper tantrums, to be fearful, to have eating problems, to have difficulty in attaining bladder control, and to be prone to accidents. These problems are likely to occur because the mothers are preoccupied with themselves or lack the energy to establish the mutual activation and the mutual regulation that characterizes a healthy mother-child relationship. Without these supporting and regulating relationships, the child does not have the enforcement necessary to inhibit impulses or an opportunity to practice, explore, and separate from his mother.

Since the depressed mother is not able to establish mutual relationships, she, likewise, is not able to communicate meaningfully with her child. She cannot function as a role model or teach her child how to communicate internal and external relationship experiences. As Weissman (1972) has shown, many depressed mothers are particularly hostile toward their child and this hostility frequently takes the form of irritability. Such irritability does not encourage a means for open, healthy, communicative relationships.

In some cases, depressed mothers have excessive concerns about their children which tends to make the child uneasy about his own abilities and thus afraid to separate and risk meeting the world. Often the mothers communicate their fears concerning the world to the child who in turn sees the world as a fearful place; one in which he is quite vulnerable.

School Age

As the child moves from the preschool period to school age, the mother's tasks change. She assumes the role of the purveyor of culture and a facilitator for peer interactions. Teaching at this time becomes more of an indirect modeling process rather than a didactic interchange. With the growth of the child's cognitive capacities, the mother, as well as other family members, becomes more like a role model for whom the child can imitate.

As a model, the depressed mother communicates her mood, her isolation, her fears of the world, and her hostility toward the child. The lack of attention and interest does not enable the child to get the support, the guidance, and the reinforcement needed in selecting friends, dealing with school, and being a social person. Grunebaum et al. (1978), in a study of schizophrenic, depressed, and well mothers, and their school aged children, found the children of depressed mothers to have greater cognitive difficulties, in certain areas, than the children of the schizophrenic and well mothers.

The child, at this age, feels an acute sense of deprivation from the mother's lack of disinterest and often feels that this is due to something that they have or have not done. Serious difficulties arise because the child assumes the responsibility for the state of his mother. When the child attempts to be different, to change, or to reach mother, the child feels frustrated and worthless because the mother greets his attempts with further withdrawal, more hostility, or scolds him as being a demanding child.

The scope of this article does not extend to the adolescent period. However, further difficulties related to separation are seen in this stage of development as well.

PREVENTION

Definition and Role in Mother-Child Relationship

Primary prevention refers to measures to avert the appearance of a disease. Secondary prevention refers to early diagnosis and prompt treatment to shorten the course of the illness, reduce symptoms, limit sequelae and minimize contagion. It is necessary to conceptualize prevention in terms of the dyadic nature of the mother-child relationship. The very basis of primary prevention is the ability to predict the occurrence of some type of mental disturbance subsequent to specific events, states, or behaviors. Our present state of knowledge concerning depression does not allow us to have this ability. Therefore, we may not be able to prevent the maternal depression. However, it is primary prevention for the child if we are able to detect depression in the mother and through biochemical, environmental manipulation, or psychotherapeutic means treat the depression; thereby enhancing the effective availability of the mother to her child. Such availability will enable her to be more responsive to her crying infant, or to her preschooler experiencing anxiety in a new situation, or to her school age child who has just done poorly on an exam for which he studied very hard.

Treatment Strategies

There is no question that the most important aspect of secondary prevention for the dyad is detection and treatment of the depression in the mother. The detection is not usually going to be done by the psychiatrist or psychologist, but by the pediatrician, visiting nurse, and personnel who staff well baby clinics. The first issue is to heighten the awareness of these front line people to the prevalence and effects of the problem. Well baby care is not routine care, but it can make critical contributions to the emotional and physical health of the mother and child. When a child is brought into the office, it is essential for the pediatrician or nurse to inquire into the psychological well-being of the mother, the nature of the mother-child interaction and the role of the father. Direct questioning of the mother is often to no avail and to perform a mental status examination on her would be inappropriate. It is important to start with the child (of any age). After listening to the issues or questions regarding the child, this behavior or state is presented as having effects on the parent. This opens the way for maternal feelings to be discussed and information about their moods, daily life, habits, etc. to be obtained. The symptoms of depression described in the section titled "Definition" should be investigated with a special eye to duration so that an evaluation of the presence of a transient state or more persistent mood disturbance can be made. Often there is much shame and guilt and concern whether or not they are being good mothers. These emotions should be discussed frankly and openly. Some women regard their depression as normal and would, therefore, not discuss it. An explanation that it is not normal is essential. Since hostility has been found as a prominent feature of depressed women, questions concerning anger towards their children and methods of discipline or punishment are needed. A comment such as "that behavior must frustrate you or get you angry" followed by a question such as "what do you do when you get angry or frustrated with your child?" will give the parents opportunity to talk about how they feel. They usually respond well to this technique.

If depression is found, the degree of depression, its effect on the mother's life and its direct effect on the child needs to be quickly assessed. With moderate to severe depression, tricyclic antidepressants may be of great help. Remember, however, medication alone will not solve the relationship problems. Symptomatic improvement may allow mother to assume a care taking function. Help from father, other relatives, visiting nurses, social workers may be needed; even day facilities may need to be considered.

O'Brien (1981) in a three-year follow-up study of the children of manic depressive parents found that despite adequate treatment and lack of serious manic or depressive episodes, subtle impairments of emotional relationships existed between mother and child. In the symptomatic child, although they knew something was wrong with the mother, the idea that she was depressed was never discussed; in fact, rarely were affective issues dealt with in the family. This led to a variety of strange fantasies on the part of the children as to what was happening to their mother. Many children felt their mother's problems were caused by something they did or did not do, especially for children up to 8 years of age. It is necessary to explain that mommy may not be in a good mood today, but her mood is not caused by the child's behavior. The family should discuss what to do or not do when this happens. Such openness takes the secret quality away and removes the burden from the children. It gives the entire family some awareness of the mother's incapacity and enables the family to mobilize its resources to help the mother and each other in the daily confrontation with the depression.

Another difficulty found in the parents of symptomatic children was a subtle impairment in the mother to involve herself with the children and an impaired ability to communicate affection. Mothers responded only to the most outrageous behaviors. The children rarely told their mothers anything about their deeper feelings and problems. During the research, some children were seriously and overtly depressed; at the same time the mothers described them as well adjusted. This type of impairment requires the family to look at the depression and talk about it, hopefully as a prelude to opening up other areas for communication such as the children's feelings. This often requires psychotherapeutic intervention.

Children of depressed mothers are often quite sensitive to separation from their mothers or their environments. This is important for mothers to know so they can plan moves or be prepared for consequences.

In some cases, environmental manipulation may be needed such as helping to find better housing, financial assistance, and respite care. Many depressed mothers are quite isolated, and group experiences, either of a community nature or in a clinic setting, are often helpful in providing support, ventilation, and social outlets.

It is easy to understand how depressed mothers are caught in a vicious cycle. At a time when such mothers need support from their husbands, the child becomes demanding and difficult to manage, and the husband becomes critical of her ability to be a mother and a wife. This cycle must be broken by a combination of means; educational, environmental, manipulation, and psychotherapeutic. Above all, care takers must know maternal depression is there and be sensitive to the evident manifestations of the disturbance to both the mother and the child.

REFERENCES

Anthony, E. J. A clinical evaluation of children with psychotic parents. *American Journal of Psychiatry*, 1969, *126*, 177-184.

Brown, G., Bhrolchain, M., and Harris, T. Social class and psychiatric disturbance among women in an urban population. *Sociology*, 1976, *9*, 225-254.

Ekdahl, M., Rice, E., and Schmidt, W. Children of parents hospitalized for mental illness. *American Journal of Public Health*, 1962, *52*, 428-435.

Grunebaum, H., Cohler, B., Kauffman, C., and Gallant, D. Children of depressed and schizophrenic mothers. *Child Psychiatry and Human Development*, 1978, *8*, 219-228.

Kendell, R., Wainwright, S., Hailey, A. et al. The influence of childbirth on psychiatric morbidity. *Psychological Medicine*, 1976, *6*, 297-302.

Kestenbaum, C., Kron, L., and Decina, P. The children of bipolar patients clinical features. Presented at the American Psychiatry Association Meeting New Orleans, 1981 (unpublished).

McKnew, D., Cytryn, L., Efron, A., et al. Offspring of patients with affective disorders. *British Journal of Psychiatry*, 1979, *134*, 148-152.

Moss, P., and Plewis, I. Mental distress in mothers of pre-school children in inner London. *Psychological Medicine*, 1977, *7*, 641-652.

O'Brien, J., Dabbs, E., Malin, S. et al. Three years follow-up study of the children of manic depressive parents. Presented at the American Academy of Child Psychiatry Meeting Chicago, 1981 (unpublished).

O'Connell, R., Mayo, J., and O'Brien, J. Children of bipolar manic depressives. In J. Mendlewicz and B. Shopsin (Eds.), *Genetic aspects of affective illness*. New York: Spectrum Publications, 1979.

Orvaschel, H., Weissman, M., Padian, N., and Lowe, T. L. Assessing psychopathology in children of psychiatrically disturbed parents: A pilot study. *Journal of the American Academy of Child Psychiatry*, 1981, *20*, 112-122.

Rutter, M. *Children of sick parents*. London: Oxford University Press, 1966.

Sanders, L. Issues in early mother-child interaction. *Journal of the American Academy of Child Psychiatry*, 1964, *2*, 141-166.

Weissman, M., Paykel, E., and Klerman, G. The depressed woman as mother. *Social Psychiatry*, 1972, *7*, 98-108.

Welner, Z., Welner, A., McCrary, M. and Leonard, M. A. Psychopathology in children of inpatients with depression. *Journal of Nervous and Mental Diseases*, 1977, *164*, 408-413.

Wolkind, S., Lajicek, E., and Ghodsian, M. Continuities in maternal depression. *International Journal of Family Psychiatry*, 1980, *1*, 167-181.

Zax, M., Sameroff, A., and Babigan, H. Birth outcomes in the offspring of mentally disordered women. *American Journal of Orthopsychiatry*, 1977, *47*, 218-230.

EPIDEMIOLOGY

The Epidemiology
of Depression in Young Children

Helen Orvaschel, PhD

ABSTRACT. Epidemiologic data provide information on the distribution of a disorder in the population and identify the risk factors associated with that disorder. True estimates of prevalence and incidence can be obtained only by measuring the extent to which a disorder is present in the population at risk. There is currently very little direct information available on the epidemiology of depression in young children. This paper reviews the reasons for this dearth of information which include: (1) controversies regarding the appropriateness of the diagnosis of depression in young children and (2) related delays in the development of necessary assessment techniques. Also presented are the data available which relate to this subject and provide insights on the extent of this problem for young children.

For many individuals the term epidemiology is associated with infectious diseases and allied with the study of epidemics. The epidemiology of chronic diseases such as heart disease, cancer, and psychiatric disorders is equally important, but less frequently considered by those working in other disciplines. The field of epide-

Dr. Orvaschel is Assistant Professor in the Department of Psychiatry, Yale University School of Medicine. Reprint requests to: Depression Research Unit, 904 Howard Avenue, Suite 2A, New Haven, CT 06519-1191.

This review was supported, in part, by Research Grant #NIMH 5 U01 MH34224 and #1-R01-MH28274.

miology in general is concerned with how a disease or disorder is distributed in a population and attempts to identify the determinants or risk factors for that disorder (MacMahon and Pugh, 1970).

Epidemiologic data also provide the information necessary for the planning and evaluation of service and treatment programs by obtaining rates of the prevalence and incidence of disorders. Prevalence is a measure of the number of individuals who have a particular disorder at a specific point in time. Incidence is a measure of the new occurrences of a disorder and is therefore more valuable for identifying causal factors.

In order to obtain true estimates of the prevalence and incidence of a disorder, one must measure the extent to which the disorder is present in the population at risk for the disorder. If the disorder of interest is depression and the population of concern is children between the ages of 4 and 8, then a measure of prevalence could be obtained only if a representative sample of this population was assessed for the presence of that disorder. Incidence could be estimated by reevaluating the sample at subsequent points in time and assessing the occurrence of new cases of depression.

Estimating the prevalence or incidence of depression in children cannot be determined from treated populations alone, since many children are never referred for treatment. In addition, treated groups generally represent a biased sample of those actually affected. Children may be more commonly referred for acting-out behavior accompanying their depression or for more severe cases of depression. Socio-demographic variables also influence who receives treatment as does the sex of the child. In order to avoid the biases inherent in clinical samples, estimates of the prevalence of depression in children should be measured in community or school samples of children in the appropriate age groups.

Historical Perspective

The types of data ascertained in psychiatric epidemiology have generally reflected the technological status as well as the theoretical orientation in which the field of psychiatry has operated at a given point in time. Early epidemiologic studies in adult psychiatry concentrated on measure of overall emotional distress (Langner, 1962; Srole et al., 1962; Leighton et al., 1963). This reflected the unitary concept of mental health at the time, as well as the unavailability of reliable measures of psychiatric disorders (Weissman and Klerman,

1978). The use of symptom inventories and factor analytic techniques began to move the field away from a unitary disease concept but still avoided the measurement of specific diagnoses.

A number of developments in psychiatry during the past decade have affected epidemiologic research. The introduction of specific diagnostic criteria such as the Research Diagnostic Criteria (RDC) (Spitzer et al., 1978), the Feighner criteria (Feighner et al., 1972) and more recently the DSM III criteria (APA, 1980) have helped to improve diagnostic reliability by operationalizing the symptoms necessary for specific categories of disorder. These criteria systems led, in turn, to the development of structured psychiatric interviews such as the Schedule for Affective Disorders and Schizophrenia (Spitzer and Endicott, 1978), the Present State Exam (Wing et al., 1974), the Renard Interview (Helzer et al., 1981), and the Diagnostic Interview Schedule (Robins et al., 1981), which reduced the information variance in diagnosis, thereby further improving diagnostic reliability (Endicott and Spitzer, 1978).

Child Psychiatric Epidemiology

Structured interviews have now been used successfully in both clinical and epidemiologic research in adult psychiatry (Weissman and Myers, 1980). Research in child psychiatry has lagged behind that of adult psychiatry, in part, because of the lack of a theoretical consensus on diagnosis and the related delays in the development of appropriate assessment techniques. Controversy in the field still exists regarding the appropriateness of categorizing child psychopathology and even greater disagreement exists about how symptoms should be grouped in the various criteria systems.

Few investigators have attempted to interview young children directly, relying instead on information from parents or teachers and reporting results of global impairment rather than discrete disorders. Jones (1977) reported that 4% of a community sample of four year olds and 8% of a community sample of seven year olds were found to be clinically disturbed when a global rating of psychopathology was used. From these data, however, there is no way of knowing what proportion of the children were suffering from an affective disorder. Similarly, Earls (1980) found that 11% of his community sample of three year olds had behavior problems. While frequently rated items included unhappy mood, dependency, worries, and poor peer relations, the prevalence of a depressive disorder was not assessed. Rutter et al. (1976) reported a 6-7% prevalence of psychiatric disorders in his community sample of 10-11 year olds. He also noted that many of the behavioral disturbances manifested at that age could probably have been detected in early childhood. Little depression was found in this study, but again it was not systematically assessed.

Evidence for Childhood Depression

Before there could be an epidemiology of childhood depression, psychiatry had first to acknowledge that the disorder could be present in young children. Early studies that provided direction in this area reported evidence which suggested that depression or emotional distress in mothers had an adverse affect on their children and that mothers with young children were particularly vulnerable to emotional distress (Weissman et al., 1972; Rolf and Garmezy, 1974; Weintraub et al., 1975; Richman, 1976; Moss and Plewis, 1977). While more research is needed on the consequences to children of poor mental health in their mothers, preliminary findings indicate that children from such families are more likely to suffer from emotional problems and depression (Munro, 1966; Jacobson et al., 1975; Welner et al., 1977).

The concept of a depressive disorder in young children is fairly recent and the controversy is still not yet over. While no one has argued that depression as an affect is not clearly evident in children, the recognition of depression as a syndrome or disorder of childhood has had an uphill battle. The terms masked depression or depressive equivalents have been offered as alternatives to a diagnosis of depression in children (Rie, 1966; Cytryn and McKnew, 1972; Lesse, 1977). Clinicians argued that manifestations of depression that resemble adult symptomatology do not occur in children. Instead, they suggested that children who are rebellious, disobedient, hypochondriacal, destructive, irritable, hyperactive, or have problems in school are expressing depressive equivalents (Burks and Harrison, 1962; Toolan, 1962; Hollon, 1970; Brandes, 1971).

Despite these previously held positions, current research in child psychiatry has shown that depression as a syndrome is found in young children and that it can be reliably diagnosed on the basis of specific symptom clusters. The concept of masked depression has been relinquished by its major proponents (Cytryn et al., 1979). While agreement has not yet been established on which symptoms should be used to constitute the clinical picture of childhood depression, many investigators view it to be similar to the adult depressive syndrome and use RDC or DSM III as diagnostic criteria (Shulterbrandt and Raskin, 1977). Developments in assessment techniques and the recent availability of structured psychiatric interviews for use with children are beginning to provide the tools necessary for obtaining the appropriate epidemiologic data (Orvaschel et al., 1980a; Orvaschel et al., 1980b).

Epidemiology of Depression

For the reasons mentioned above, there is a paucity of epidemiologic information on childhood depression. Studies that provide data related to this subject do exist, although the samples are, with few exceptions, not representative of the general population.

In a study of children referred to a neuropsychiatric unit, Carlson and Cantwell (1979) evaluated 102 children between the ages of 7-17 years. While 60% of these children presented with symptoms of depression, withdrawal, and suicidal ideation, only 27% were considered to have an affective disorder. The sub-group with depression included a small number of children under the age of 12. Another study of pre-pubertal depressive disorder reports that about 15% of their patients are age 8 or under (Puig-Antich and Tabrizi, 1981). Interestingly, a frequently accompanying symptom of the depressive disorder in this younger population is separation anxiety.

More relevant to epidemiologic data are two recent studies reported by Kashani et al. In the first study, 103 children between the ages of 7-12 who were selected from a family practice clinic and from medical center birth records were evaluated. While the symptom of sadness was found present in 17.4% of the sample, a prevalence of 1.9% was reported for those meeting DSM III criteria of depression (Kashani and Simonds, 1979). In a second study, Kashani et al. (1981a) examined 100 children between 7-12 years of age who were admitted to a pediatric ward. They found 7% of the children met criteria for depression. Three of the children who were depressed were age 8 or less.

As is evident, estimates of the prevalence of depression differ as a function of the population studied. Prevalence rates ranging from .14% to 59% have been reported for childhood depression, but the samples on which these estimates were made varied in age, assessment instruments and criteria used, source of information, and type of sample studied (Kashani et al., 1981b).

The only community data of childhood depression were recently reported by Lefkowitz and Tesiny (1981). They studied 3020 pre-pubertal children drawn from the 3rd, 4th, and 5th grades. Depression was assessed using a Peer Nomination Inventory of Depression (PNID) which had been previously standardized on classroom children. Children were categorized as depressed if they scored two standard deviations above the mean. A 5.2% prevalence rate for depression was reported for the overall sample, but for children age 8.5 or less the prevalence of depression was 4.76% for females and 6.98% for males. This study did not use DSM III diagnostic criteria, nor did it obtain clinical confirmation by direct interviews with the children, but it does represent a first step in obtaining non-biased rates of childhood depression in the population.

Conclusions

Obtaining epidemiologic data on the prevalence of childhood depression has had many obstacles to overcome. The concept of a depressive disorder in children, with age appropriate symptoms and developmental considerations in assessment, has not yet been agreed upon. Despite these obstacles, evidence has been reported for the presence of this disorder in young children and studies of the prevalence of childhood depression are beginning to appear. With the advent of such epidemiologic studies, we will have a greater opportunity to identify associated risk factors which may be specific to depression, estimate the need for treatment in the child population, and hopefully initiate prevention strategies for children at risk for this disorder.

REFERENCES

American Psychiatric Association. *Diagnostic and Statistical Manual of Mental Disorders, 3rd ed. (DSM III)*. Washington, D.C., 1980.

Brandes, N. S. A discussion of depression in children and adolescents. *Clinical Pediatrics,* 1971, *10,* 470-475.

Burks, H. L., and Harrison, S. I. Aggressive behavior as a means of avoiding depression. *American Journal of Orthopsychiatry,* 1962, *32,* 416-422.

Carlson, G. A., and Cantwell, D. P. A survey of depressive symptoms in a child and adolescent psychiatric population. *Journal of the American Academy of Child Psychiatry,* 1979, *18,* 587-599.

Cytryn, L., and McKnew, D. H. Proposed classification of childhood depression. *American Journal of Psychiatry,* 1972, *129,* 149-155.

Cytryn, L., McKnew, D. H., and Bunney, W. E. Diagnosis of depression in children. *American Journal of Psychiatry,* 1979, *137,* 12-25.

Earls, F. The prevalence of behavior problems in three-year old children. *Archives of General Psychiatry,* 1980, *37,* 1153-1157.

Endicott, J., and Spitzer, R. L. A diagnostic interview: The schedule for affective disorders and schizophrenia. *Archives of General Psychiatry*, 1978, *35*, 837-844.

Feighner, J. P., Robins, E., Guze, S. B. et al. Diagnostic criteria for use in psychiatric research. *Archives of General Psychiatry*, 1972, *26*, 57-63.

Helzer, J. E., Robins, L. N., Croughan, J. L. et al. Reliability and procedural validity of the Renard Diagnostic Interview as used by physicians and lay interviewers. *Archives of General Psychiatry,* in press.

Hollon, T. H. Poor school performance as a symptom of masked depression in children and adolescents. *American Journal of Psychotherapy,* 1970, *24,* 258-263.

Jacobson, S., Fasman, J., and DeMascio, A. Deprivation in the childhood of depressed women. *Journal of Nervous and Mental Disease,* 1975, *166,* 5-14.

Jones, F. H. The Rochester Adaptive Behavior Inventory: A parallel series of instruments for assessing social competence during early and middle childhood and adolescence. In J. S. Strauss, H. M. Babigian, and M. Roff (Eds.), *The origins and course of psychopathology.* New York: Plenum Press, 1977.

Kashani, J. H., and Simonds, J. F. The incidence of depression in children. *American Journal of Psychiatry,* 1979, *136,* 1203-1205.

Kashani, J. H., Barbero, G. T., and Bolander, F. D. Depression in hospitalized pediatric patients. *Journal of the American Academy of Child Psychiatry,* 1981, *20,* 123-134. (a)

Kashani, J. H., Husain, A., Shekim, W. D. et al. Current perspectives on childhood depression: An overview. *Journal of the American Academy of Child Psychiatry,* 1981, *138,* 143-153. (b)

Langner, T. S. A 22 item screening score of psychiatric symptoms indicating impairment. *Journal of Health and Human Behavior,* 1962, *3,* 269-276.

Leighton, D. C., Harding, J. S., Macklin, D. B. et al. Psychiatric findings of the Sterling County study. *American Journal of Psychiatry,* 1963, *119,* 1021-1026.

Lefkowitz, M. M., and Tesiny, E. P. The epidemiology of depression in normal children. Presented at the American Association for the Advancement of Science, Toronto, 1981.

Lesse, S. Masked depression and depressive equivalents. *Psychopharmacology Bulletin,* 1977, *13,* 68-70.

MacMahon, B., and Pugh, T. F. *Epidemiology: Principles and methods.* Boston: Little, Brown and Co., 1970.

Moss, P., and Plewis, I. Mental distress in mothers of pre-school children in Inner London. *Psychological Medicine,* 1977, *7,* 641-652.

Munro, A. Some familial and social factors in depressive illness. *British Journal of Psychiatry,* 1966, *112,* 429-441.

Orvaschel, H., Sholomskas, D., and Weissman, M. M. *The assessment of psychopathology and behavioral problems in children: A review of scales suitable for epidemiologic and clinical research (1967-1978).* NIMH, Series AN No. 1, DHHS Publication No. (ADM) 80-1037, Washington, D.C., 1980.(a)

Orvaschel, H., Sholomskas, D., and Weissman, M. M. Assessing children in psychiatric epidemiologic studies. In F. Earls (Ed.), *Monographs in pyschosocial epidemiology, I. Studies of Children.* New York: Prodist 1980.(b)

Puig-Antich, J., and Tabrizi, M. A. Personal communication, September 1981.

Richman, N. Depression in mothers of preschool children. *Journal of Child Psychology and Psychiatry,* 1976, *17,* 75-78.

Rie, H. E. Depression in childhood—A survey of some pertinent contributions. *Journal of the American Academy of Child Psychiatry,* 1966, *5,* 653-685.

Robins, L., Helzer, J., Croughan, J. et al. The NIMH Diagnostic Interview Schedule, Version 3. National Institute of Mental Health, ADM-42-12-79, 1981.

Rolf, J. E., and Garmezy, N. The school performance of children vulnerable to behavior pathology. In D. F. Ricks, T. Alexander, and M. Roff (Eds.), *Life history research in psychopathology,* Vol. 3, Minnesota: University of Minnesota Press, 1974.

Rutter, M., Tizard, J., Yule, W. et al. Isle of Wight Studies, 1964-1974. *Psychological Medicine,* 1976, *6,* 313-332.

Shulterbrandt, J. G., and Raskin, A. *Depression in children—Diagnosis, treatment and conceptual models.* New York: Raven Press, 1977.

Spitzer, R. L., and Endicott, J. Schedule for affective disorders and schizophrenia. National Institute of Mental Health, Clinical Research Branch, Collaborative Program on the Psychobiology of Depression, Third Edition, May 1978.

Spitzer, R. L., Endicott, J., and Robins E. Research diagnostic criteria: Rationale and reliability. *Archives of General Psychiatry,* 1978, *35,* 773-782.

Srole, L., Langer, T. S., Michael, S. T. et al. *Mental health in the metropolis: The Midtown Manhattan study, Vol. 1:* New York: McGraw-Hill, 1962.

Toolan, J. M. Depression in children and adolescents. *American Journal of Orthopsychiatry,* 1962, *32,* 404-414.

Weintraub, S., Neale, J. M., and Liebert, D. E. Teacher ratings of children vulnerable to psychopathology. *American Journal of Orthopsychiatry,* 1975, *45,* 839-845.

Weissman, M. M., Paykel, E. S., and Klerman, G. L. The depressed woman as a mother. *Social Psychiatry,* 1972, *7,* 98-108.

Weissman, M. M., and Myers, J. K. Psychiatric disorders in a U.S. community. *Acta Psychiatric Scandinavia,* 1980, *62,* 99-111.

Weissman, M. M., and Klerman, G. L. Epidemiology of mental disorders. *Archives of General Psychiatry,* 1978, *35,* 705-712.

Welner, Z., Welner, A., and McCrary, M. D. et al. Psychopathology in children of inpatients with depression—A controlled study. *Journal of Nervous and Mental Disease,* 1977, *164,* 408-413.

Wing, J. K., Cooper, J. E., and Sartorius, N. *The measurement and classification of psychiatric symptoms.* London: Cambridge University Press, 1974.

ADVANCED RESEARCH

Future Trends in the Study and Treatment of Depression in Young Children

Theodore A. Petti, MD

ABSTRACT. The controversy over the existence of depression in children has abated and the maturation process of further delineation of the disorder has begun. Future advances in understanding, identifying and treating young dysphoric children will be based on the ongoing work described in this journal issue. Suggested areas where these thrusts will appear include the early identification of depressed young children, delineation of the frequency and situations where the depression occurs, primary mental health prevention, more comprehensive therapeutic interventions and determination of biological correlates. Samplings of these "goodies" are provided.

This issue of the *Journal of Children in Contemporary Society* provides an overview of depression in young children and insights into issues as to how dysphoria presents itself at various age levels and environmental settings. A blossoming of related research, clinical reports and descriptions of therapeutic interventions can be expected to appear in the next five years as professionals involved with the care and treatment of young children devote more time and attention to childhood depression.

Dr. Petti is Assistant Professor of Child Psychiatry, University of Pittsburgh School of Medicine and Director, Section on Children and Youth, Office of Education and Regional Programming, Western Psychiatric Institute and Clinic, University of Pittsburgh, Pittsburgh, Pennsylvania 15261.

Early Identification of Depressed Young Children

Earlier identification and detection efforts at primary mental health prevention, and more specific intervention strategies at all levels of prevention and care are areas with the greatest potential for future progress toward decreasing the disability associated with depression in young children. The present state of assessing the depressive state, the contributing factors to its development and finally the relation of its assessment to treatment have been described throughout this issue. We can expect, for example, investigators such as Kashani and Associates to begin systematic studies into the nature of depressive disorders in preschool children, a heretofore unexplored area. These efforts combined with those ongoing for older children will lead to more precise diagnoses, greater research efforts and a new burst of useful knowledge through the facilitation of communication between professionals.

A natural progression of this work is the determination of how frequently depression occurs in young children, particularly with regard to different settings. This is of critical importance to the task of systematically understanding conditions which lead to depression and to types of environments or interventions that tend to decrease the chances that the depression will occur. Orvaschel (1982) has addressed many essential issues that need to be considered before epidemiologic studies can be truly useful in identifying risk factors and instituting prevention measures. Epidemiology has been designated as a major area for research in mental health for the next several years, thus results from such studies can be anticipated.

The issues related to the effects of depressed parents on their young offspring is an important aspect of epidemiologic and clinical work. O'Brien (1982) calls on professionals to be more aware of the impact of the depressed mother and cites the limited, but growing attention to this area (Kestenbaum et al., 1979; McKnew et al., 1979; Orvaschel et al., 1981). A child who manifests depressive symptoms should be an alert to look for a depressed parent who might benefit from counseling and/or medication. Moreover, as knowledge about the genetic and familial relationships of depression get teased apart and and appreciation that depressed parents often raise depressed or vulnerable children develops, the therapists of those parents will be expected to consider the effects of the illness on the children and to take the necessary steps to lessen the negative impact on them.

Several papers in this issue have described special groups of young children who often develop depressive symptoms. Cantwell and Baker (1982), for example, tie together the special vulnerability of children with a language disorder and a speech/language disorder to affective illness. They note that children with academic failure but without a formal depressive disorder had depressive symptomatology as a major component of their psychiatric problems. This group who may not be diagnosed by physicians as significantly depressed still need to be identified and the depressive component considered for treatment. Scales and interview schedules should be of assistance to the clinician for monitoring such cases. Petti (1981, 1982) portrays the linkage between learning disability, depression and hyperactive behavior. He describes the low self-esteem and feelings of having no control over their destiny that learning disabled children frequently experience.

The young child with severe burns is part of another special, vulnerable group. Stoddard and O'Connell (1982) poignantly focus our attention on the dysphoria of such children in the various stages of care. The insights derived from their work and the interest of workers in other pediatric/medical disorders (Poznanski et al., 1979; Kashani et al., 1981 a,b; Petti, 1981) should result in an expanded literature regarding primary and secondary prevention of depression in medically ill children.

Children who experience the loss of a parent or caretaker are especially prone to depression. McConville summarizes his work in understanding loss as a precipitator of depression in children and provides a model for its study within a developmental context. Continued reports that tease apart the varying responses of children to both acute and chronic stress and loss—situations believed to cause depression in adults may assist in our efforts to understand the interaction between behavior, physiologic changes and the course of childhood depression. The works of Wallerstein and Kelly (1980) provide us with more data from such a model based on children's responses to divorce and separation. Such children develop both short-term grief or acute dysphoria (adjustment disorders with depression and/or anxiety) and longer term dysthymic or major depressive reactions. The approaches they employ may be prototypical of identification programs for the future.

The abused child may also be among the most vulnerable to depression (Irwin et al., 1981). Such children may be difficult to assess and non-verbal techniques may be of great utility. The work of Cytryn and McKnew (1974) and Portner (1982) suggest that attending to the fantasy of young children can assist in identifying those at risk for problems associated with depression and possibly serve as a means of longitudinally monitoring the course and process of the disorder, and the effects of intervention. This is poignantly illustrated in the treatment of psychoanalysts working with young children (Lopez and Kliman, 1979; Cohen, 1980).

Primary Prevention

The most significant advances in the next decade may well occur in the area of primary mental health prevention. Programs such as the Interpersonal Cognitive or Social Problem Solving (ICPS) skills training for preschoolers (Shure and Spivack, 1978), the Primary Mental Health Project (Cowen, 1980) for young school age children and Channel Specific Perceptual Stimulation (Silver and Hagin, 1972; Arnold et al., 1977) are potential models.

The Shure and Spivack program has demonstrated that four and five-year-old children differ in their abilities to think through and solve interpersonal problems and that children who were more capable of solving such problems were better adjusted socially than the children who were not so adept. They found that young children can be trained in ICPS skills by teachers or parents and that those who improved most in social adjustment also improve in the skills training. The ICPS skills taught included consequential thinking (e.g., what happens next when you grab a toy from a peer), causal thinking (i.e., linking one interpersonal event to a previous one to understand what might have contributed to an action), sensitivity to interpersonal problems, and alternative thinking (i.e., conceptualizing alternative solutions to problems). This is done through a series of ten 20-minute sessions of games and dialogues carried out by nursery school teachers or parents. It includes the teaching of words such as ''or'' and ''maybe.''

Since children with learning and academic problems are vulnerable to developing significant dysphoria, work in lessening the deficits in learning disabled children can be of tremendous value in decreasing the development of depression in children. Arnold (1977) has demonstrated in a controlled study how specific perceptual deficits can be trained out of first grade children and that children receiving this special training did significantly better in learning and social adjustment that did similarly disabled children who had received tutoring or "special attention" for equivalent periods of time.

Thus programs which address the social, cognitive and learning related needs of children do have a positive impact on children and have great potential for decreasing the development of hopelessness, helplessness, low self-esteem and depression.

Secondary Prevention and Treatment

The predominant form of therapy of children with depression has been conducted by psychoanalytically or psychodynamically oriented professionals. Successes in psychoanalytic treatment of young, depressed children (Cohen, 1980) are still being reported. This approach, though still important in understanding how the individual child organizes depressive constructs, is being supplemented and may ultimately be replaced by multimodal, shorter term, less expensive treatment.

Research into treatment of depressive children looms invitingly over the horizon. The use of antidepressant medication, of course, will be one of the areas of greatest interest. Imipramine (Tofranil) has been the most commonly used drug of this type and it has been found to be effective in treating a number of symptoms commonly related to depression (Petti, 1983). Open studies have been very positive regarding its efficacy with depressed children. Weinberg and Associates (1973) have detailed the high frequency of dysphoria in children with academic and behavior problems in the early school grades. Children who met research criteria for depression were found to show a statistically significant response to antidepressant medication.

Generally, therapeutic interventions are not accepted as efficacious unless an overwhelming body of evidence supports such a conclusion and/or double-blind controlled studies with placebo show statistically positive results. A number of issues, including the fact that the depression of young children may be dissimilar in etiology, physiology and presentation, call for a re-examination of the appropriateness of the large group design to the study of therapeutic interventions (Petti and Conners, 1981). Thus far only one double blind pilot study which includes young school children, has demonstrated that imipramine is more effective than placebo (Petti and Law, 1982). However, suggestions have been made from recent studies that children need to reach certain anti-depressant plasma levels in order for the drug to work (Weller et al., 1981; Puig-Antich and Perel, 1981). If true, this can be an exciting breakthrough in providing greater safety and control in using a highly effective agent to treat very disabling disorders. Problems with getting accurate and valid plasma levels of the antidepressants are being solved so this obstacle to their use is being eliminated.

Non-biological methods of treatment will not be lost and will continue to be of importance in this decade. A shift from the long-term psychoanalytic, several times weekly, approach to shorter term, weekly psychodynamic/behavioral/cognitive therapies is likely to occur as interventions directed specifically to target symptoms of depression get developed. The literature to date has been described elsewhere (Petti, 1981, 1982). Representative examples may provide a taste for such approaches.

Many non-hospitalized, depressed children manifest aggressive behavior—perhaps as a reaction to their sense of helplessness and inability to cope. An effective behavioral/cognitive approach in helping such youngsters has been described (Camp et al., 1977). Aggressive second grade boys (ages 6 to 8 years) were taught to "think aloud" and to develop verbal mediation skills and prosocial behaviors in response to problematic situations.

Likewise, teaching disturbed children more adaptive and alternative behaviors to take the place of fighting, withdrawing, obsessing and so on have been highly successful. For example, social skills training has been used to help aggressive (Bornstein et al., 1980) and withdrawn children (Bornstein et al., 1977) function better in various settings. Targeted behaviors included making eye contact, smiling when being complimented, requesting new behavior from peers or others and increasing their duration of speech. A bibliography of the behavioral treatment of the "hyperkinetic behavior syndrome" (Reatig, 1980) should provide help to those interested in learning more about this type approach.

Multimodal, comprehensive treatment of addressing the various contributing factors to the development and maintenance of depression in the young child—home, school, community, intropsychic, physiologic, cognitive and/or coordinating the relevant interventions may well prove to be the least expensive and most efficacious therapy in decreasing the depression and preventing further disability. Models and case studies of this approach have been described elsewhere (Petti, 1981, 1982a; McConville, 1982).

New Frontiers

Biological correlates of dysphoria are just now being studied and show promise for providing breakthroughs in the assessment, management and understanding of depressed children. For example, two approaches with adults, which have the capacity to differentiate certain types of depressed from non-depressed individuals, are the dexamethasone suppression test (DST) and all night EEG sleep studies (polysomnography). Both have been used to some extent with children.

The results of polysomnography with depressed children treated with antidepressant medication have been reported (Kupfer et al., 1979). A report describing the polysomnographic records of normal children is in progress and the results should be useful in understanding the differences found in sleep records regarding Rapid Eye Movement and related polysomnographic parameters of depressed children. The DST on the other hand is a simpler, less expensive test which measures the individual's response to a dose of dexamethasone, a steroid medication. The normal adult or child would respond by having a suppression of their cortisol secretion. But moderately depressed individuals fail to show the normal suppression response and have a "breakthrough" and continued secretion of cortisol. Moreover, those patients who respond to treatment or show a spontaneous recovery have their DST revert back to the normal suppression response. Poznanski (1981) has found that many depressed children, as defined by research criteria, fail to demonstrate the normal suppression response. Supporting evidence for this finding has been reported by Puig-Antich and Associates (1979). They found that in severely disturbed children, as in depressed adults, excess cortisol was produced; as with such adults, upon recovery, the cortisol production markedly decreases. This area is expected to generate a great deal of research and insights as attempts are made to demonstrate the commonality between child and adult major depressive disorders (Puig-Antich, 1980).

Summary

The advances to date concerning awareness of depressive disorders in young children, approaches to assessing and identifying the disorders, determining their frequency, understanding their presentation and nature in special groups of children, tearing apart their root causes and contributing factors, and developing more efficacious approaches to prevention and treatment should continue. In a period of dwindling resources for research and direct services, the creative capacities of the people working with young children will be stressed and tested repeatedly. The frustrations of working in such a climate, "burn out" and "learned helplessness" may be the biggest obstacle to hurdle as we strive to provide the optimal, if not at least the "good enough" climate required for vulnerable children. We can and should overcome these barriers in the coming decade. By being aware that a child is depressed and by active involvement in changing the condition, the staff working with such children and their families can protect themselves from the contagion of depression and begin to feel more effective in their work.

REFERENCES

Arnold, L. E., Barnebey, N., McManus, J., Smeltzer, A., Conrad, A., Winer, G., and Desgranges, L. Prevention by specific perceptual remediation for vulnerable first graders. *Archives of General Psychiatry,* 1977, *34:*1279-1296.

Bornstein, M. R., Bellack, A. S., & Hersen, M. Social skills training for unassertive children: A multiple-baseline analysis. *Journal of Applied Behavioral Analysis,* 1977, *10:*183-195.

Bornstein, M. R., Bellack, A. S., & Hersen, M. Social skills training for highly aggressive children in an inpatient psychiatric setting. *Behavior Modification,* 1980, *4:*173-186.

Camp, B. W., Bloom, G. E., Herbert, F., & Van Doorninck, W. J. "Think aloud": A program for developing self-control in young aggressive boys. *Journal of Abnormal Child Psychology,* 1977, *5:*157-169.

Cantwell, D. P., & Baker, L. Depression in children with speech, language and learning disorders. *Journal of Children in Contemporary Society,* 1982, *15*(1).

Cohen, D. J. Constructive and reconstructive activities in the analysis of a depressed child. In A. J. Solnit, R. S. Eissler, A. Freud, M. Kris, & P. B. Neubauer (Eds.), *The psychoanalytic study of the child,* Vol. 35. New Haven: Yale University Press, 1980.

Cowen, E. L. The primary mental health project: Yesterday, today and tomorrow. *The Journal of Special Education,* 1980, *14:*133-154.

Cytryn, L., & McKnew, D. H., Jr. Factors influencing the changing clinical expression of the depressive process in children. *American Journal of Psychiatry,* 1974, *131:*879-881.

Irwin, E., Portner, E., Elmer, E., & Petti, T. A. Joyless children: The effects of abuse over time. Paper presented at the International Congress of the American Society of Psychopathology of Expression, Boston, April 1981.

Kashani, J. H., Barbero, G. J., & Bolander, F. D. Depression in hospitalized pediatric patients. *Journal of the American Academy of Child Psychiatry,* 1981, *20:*123-134. (a)

Kashani, J. H., Venzki, R., & Miller, E. A. Depression in children admitted to hospital for orthopedic procedures. *British Journal of Psychiatry,* 1981, *138:*21-25. (b)

Kestenbaum, C. J. Children at risk for manic-depressive illness. *The American Journal of Psychiatry,* 1979, *136:*1206-1207.

Kupfer, D. J., Coble, P., Kane, J., Petti, T., & Conners, C. K. Imipramine and EEG sleep in children with depressive symptoms. *Psychopharmacology,* 1979, *60:*117-123.

Lopez, T., & Kliman, G. W. Memory, reconstruction and mourning in the analysis of a 4-year-old child. In A. J. Solnit, R. S. Eissler, A. Freud, M. Kris, & P. B. Neubauer (Eds.), *The psychoanalytic study of the child,* Vol. 34, New Haven: Yale Universities Press, 1979.

McConville, B. J. The causes and treatment of depression in young children. *Journal of Children in Contemporary Society*, 1982, *15*(2).

McKnew, D. H., Cytryn, L., Efron, A. M., Gershon, E. S., & Bunney, W. E., Jr. Offspring of patients with affective disorders. *British Journal of Psychiatry*, 1979, *134:*148-152.

O'Brien, J. D. Intervention and prevention strategies for children with depressed mothers. *Journal of Children in Contemporary Society*, 1982, *15*(2).

Orvaschel, H. The epidemiology of depression in young children. *Journal of Children in Contemporary Society*, 1982, *15*(2).

Orvaschel, H., Weissman, M. M., Padian, N., & Lowe, T. L. Assessing psychopathology in children of psychiatrically disturbed parents. *Journal of the American Academy of Child Psychiatry*, 1981, *20:*112-122.

Petti, T. A. Active treatment of childhood depression. In J. F. Clarkin & H. I. Glazer (Eds.), *Depression: Behavioral and directive intervention strategies*. New York: Garland Press, 1981(a).

Petti, T. A. Depression and withdrawal in children. In O. H. Ollendick & M. Hersen (Eds.), *Handbook of child psychopathology*, New York: Plenum Publishing Corp., 1981.(b)

Petti, T. A. Imipramine in the treatment of depressed children. In D. Cantwell & G. Carlson (Eds.), *Childhood depression*, New York: Spectrum Publications, 1983.

Petti, T. A., & Conners, C. K. Imipramine treatment of depressed children. Paper delivered at the American Academy of Child Psychiatry Annual Meeting, Dallas, October 1981.

Petti, T. A., & Law, W. Imipramine treatment of depressed children: A double-blind pilot study. *Journal of Clinical Psychopharmacology*, 1982.

Portner, E. S. Depressive themes in children's fantasies. *Journal of Children in Contemporary Society*, 1982, *15*(2).

Poznanski, E. O., Cook, S. C., & Carroll, B. J. A depression rating scale for children. *Pediatrics*, 1979, *64:*442-450.

Poznanski, E. Personal communication, 1981.

Puig-Antich, J. Affective disorders in childhood: A review and perspective. *Psychiatric Clinics of North America*, 1980, *3:*403-424.

Puig-Antich, J., Chambers, W., Halpern, F., Hanlon, C., & Sachar, E. J. Cortisol hypersecretion in prepubertal depressive illness: A preliminary report. *Psychoneuroendocrinology*, 1979, *4:*191-197.

Puig-Antich, J., & Perel, J. Personal communication, 1981.

Reatig, N. A. Proceedings of the National Institute of Mental Health Workshop on the Hyperkinetic Behavior Syndrome, 1980.

Shure, M. B., & Spivack, G. *Problem solving techniques in childrearing*. San Francisco: Jossey-Bass, 1978.

Silver, A. A., & Hagin, R. A. Profile of a first grade, A basis for preventive psychiatry. *Journal of the American Academy of Child Psychiatry*, 1972, *11:*645-674.

Stoddard, F. J., & O'Connell, K. G. Dysphoria in children with severe burns. *Journal of Children in Contemporary Society*, 1982, *15*(2).

Wallerstein, J. S., & Kelly, J. B. Surviving the breakup: How children and parents cope with divorce. Basic Books: New York, 1980.

Weinberg, W. A., Rutman, J., Sullivan, L., Penick, E. C., & Dietz, S. G. Depression in children referred to an educational diagnostic center: Diagnosis and treatment. *Pediatrics, 1973, 83:*1065-1072.

Weller, E. B., Weller, R. A., Preskorn, S. H., & Glotzbach, R. Steady-state plasma imipramine levels in prepubertal depressed children. Delivered at the American Academy of Child Psychiatry Annual Meeting, Dallas, October 1981.